Healthy Life Kitchen

Healthy Life Kitchen

Marilu Henner

with Lorin Henner

ReganBooks

An Imprint of HarperCollinsPublishers

A hardcover edition of this book was published in 2000 by ReganBooks, an imprint of HarperCollins Publishers.

HEALTHY LIFE KITCHEN. Copyright © 2000 by Marilu Henner. All rights reserved. Printed in the United States of America. No part of this book may be used or reproduced in any manner whatsoever without written permission except in the case of brief quotations embodied in critical articles and reviews. For information address HarperCollins Publishers Inc., 10 East 53rd Street, New York, NY 10022.

HarperCollins books may be purchased for educational, business, or sales promotional use. For information please write: Special Markets Department, HarperCollins Publishers Inc., 10 East 53rd Street, New York, NY 10022.

First paperback edition published 2002.

Designed by Nicola Ferguson

The Library of Congress has cataloged the hardcover edition as follows:

Henner, Marilu.
     Healthy life kitchen / Marilu Henner, with Lorin Henner.
     —1st ed.
        p.   cm.
     Includes index.
     ISBN 0-06-039364-5
     1. Nutrition. 2. Diet. 3. Cookery. I. Henner, Lorin. II. Title

RA784 .H455 2000
613.2—dc21   00-032806

ISBN 0-06-098857-6 (pbk.)

02 03 04 05 06 ❖/RRD 10 9 8 7 6 5 4 3 2 1

To everyone who has a thirst

for knowledge and a hunger

for great food

contents

acknowledgments

With thanks and love . . .

To Judith Regan, who never fails to amaze me with her intelligence, beauty, tenacity, and friendship, and her unstoppable team at Regan Books and Harper-Collins—Douglas Corcoran, Renée Iwaszkiewicz, Charles Woods, Carl Raymond, Cassie Jones, Roni Axelrod, Steven Sorrentino, and especially Paul Olsewski, who always makes the book tour such a blast.

To Mel Berger, Marc Schwartz, Sam Haskell, and Rick Bradley of the William Morris Agency, Dick Guttman and Susan Madore of Guttman & Associates, and Richard Feldstein and Barbara Barbour at Provident Financial Management.

To the fabulous Deborah Wald and her darling assistant Arturo for the cover photograph.

To my talented and beautiful sister, JoAnn Carney, for her food photography and her creative and engaging team—Kimberly Hanson, Ronnda Hamilton, Laurie Baer, Claire Harbo, Michael Negreti, and Lorraine Hart. And especially to my stepson Lorne Lieberman for his camera assistance, loving support, and tasty recipes.

To all of the chefs from my favorite restaurants, cookbooks, and especially to my website regulars who taught me to keep the recipes simple and the ingredients accessible.

To Dr. Ruth Velikovsky Sharon, the incomparable psychoanalyst, with gratitude for her insights and brilliance throughout the years.

To Brent "Magic Fingers" Strickland for his positive attitude and great smile. To Inara George, who started out the rookie on the team and became the MVP because of her warmth, poise, and grace under pressure. To Bryony Atkinson, whose perception, diligence, and dry wit are surpassed only by her foxiness. To MaryAnn Hennings, a fabulous friend and cook who always proves you can eat a lot on this program and still be a babe. To Caroline Aaron, who always adds her special brand of humor, insight, and intelligence (and now cooking expertise!). To Elizabeth Carney, my wonderful niece, whose charm, ability, and talent cannot be surpassed (and what a cook!). To my sister-in-law Lynnette Lesko Henner and her incredible parents, Steve and Loretta Lesko, for their love and support. And to my brother, Lorin, my favorite coauthor, whose concentration, research ability, writing skills, and sense of humor made this book my favorite of our five collaborations. Thank you, team, I love you all!

And, last but not least . . . the secret to a great recipe is to harmoniously combine some of nature's best ingredients. The secret to a great cookbook is this:

Preheat a good idea.

Combine a dollop each of Bryony Atkinson and Inara George.

Heat Brent Strickland slowly and steadily and allow to thicken.

Add a dash of MaryAnn Hennings to season with taste.

Pour freely a healthy dose of Caroline Aaron and allow to spice and sizzle.

Stir in as much Elizabeth Carney as you can handle.

Beat my brother, Lorin Henner, for about three months till he's completely whipped and about twelve pounds overweight (*not* from the recipes!).

Whisk a bowl of Elena Lewis and add a wholesome pinch for good measure.

Add a generous and loving heap of Donna Erickson.

Knead in my husband, Robert Lieberman, cover with moist towel, and let him rise.

Squeeze as tight as possible two little hot chili peppers, Nicky and Joey.

Tenderize and thank all.

introduction

.

I have been racking my brain for weeks now trying to figure out how to start this book. Do I start with a personal story from childhood about the smells, tastes, and emotions felt while watching Mom cook with love? My mother definitely loved us, but I don't know how much of that went into her cooking. She taught dancing in our garage and ran a beauty salon out of our kitchen, so the kitchen smell I remember most is that of perm solution. (As my uncle used to say, "As a cook, she was a very good dance teacher.")

Maybe I should begin this cookbook on a more global level. I could start with the staggering statistic that despite the fact that the average restaurant meal contains one thousand to two thousand calories and fifty to one hundred grams of fat, we are currently eating in restaurants at least four or five times a week. We are cooking at home less and less often. (Most people say they don't even know the first step to cooking healthy for their families.)

Or maybe I should start this book (as I always want to start my books) with the loudest voice possible, shouting, screaming, and declaring I LOVE THIS FOOD! Believe me, I like to be healthy and I like to be fit, but most of all, I love to eat. There is no way I could have eaten this way for the last twenty-one years if the food I ate was unappetizing and unsatisfying. Discipline can only take you so far. After a while even the most resolved among us will cave in to cravings and longings for the things we have given up. But what if we didn't have to give up our favorite foods? What if we could take recipes from our childhood or favorite cookbooks and find healthier and better-tasting ways to make them? And *what if* we ended up looking better and feeling better as a result?

. . .

When people come to my home for the first time, they usually expect something like steamed vegetables and a block of tofu. (I'm not kidding. This was actually served to me once by a well-meaning host.) I love to surprise my dinner guests by serving traditional dishes they would expect at any dinner party, except that these dishes contain nothing that is harmful to their health: no red meat, no refined sugar, no dairy products, and no chemicals. My guests are often amazed that these healthy dishes taste so much better than what they're used to. I always tell them the reason is simple: it's REAL food!

It seems so unfair to me that "health food" has a bad rap. I spoke recently at an event hosted by *Healthy Dining* where famous California chefs presented the most amazing dishes (most of them within the same guidelines as *The Total Health Makeover*). The smells and textures and colors of the food were so rich and exciting and sensual, I couldn't help but think health food is really sexy! It's funny that people think a healthy, firm, vibrant body is sexy, but they don't relate the same principles to a vegetable. (On second thought . . .)

Many people love to cook and know how rewarding it can be. They have a pretty good idea of what makes a meal healthy, but they don't bother going to the trouble because they feel it's too time consuming to prepare and clean up afterward. They end up eating a lot of fast food, takeout, and prepackaged foods instead. All of these are usually high in fats, processed flour, sugar, and/or chemicals and are almost never made from *fresh* or *live* food. Most people assume that healthy meals are more difficult and require more time to prepare than junk food. The truth is that preparing healthy food doesn't have to be more burdensome or time consuming. The trick is to design your kitchen so that healthy eating becomes simple and convenient. Many people are intimidated by recipes and preparation because their kitchens are not organized for cooking and easy cleanup.

That is why I wanted to write this book. I not only wanted to turn you on to the best recipes I've ever presented, but more importantly, to explain to you how important it is to have a Healthy Life Kitchen. A Healthy Life Kitchen eventually produces a Healthy Living you! But it's a good news–bad news story. If you're like most people, 70 percent of the contents of your kitchen right now is unhealthy and has got to go. But the good news is that there are healthy and tasty alternatives to *everything*! The transition is easier than you think. I'll show you how. Together, we will not only get rid of the health robbers in your refrigerator, freezer, and pantry, we will also look under your sink and examine the harmful chemicals in your cleaning products that may be killing you. We'll explore your kitchen top to bottom, from organizing your utensil drawer to discussing what pots and pans are best to buy. And speaking of shopping, I'm taking you to the health food store and turning you on to the best products I've discovered in my twenty-one years of total health living.

So let's strip down that kitchen of yours and literally turn it into a health factory. You're not alone. I've been there myself. If you had looked in my refrigerator before I got into health, all you would have seen were Tab, Dijon mustard, and nail polish. (Not that I was on some crazy nail polish diet. Refrigeration is a great way to keep nail polish from separating.) I've done kitchen makeovers for most of my friends. I've done them on several talk shows. I even did one at my children's school. Now it's your turn.

This book is a compilation of the best recipes from my favorite cookbooks, restaurants, website members, friends, and family. You will notice that there are no nutritional analyses for these recipes. Weighing, measuring, and/or counting calories or fat, carbohydrate, and protein grams in my food stopped being a priority when I gave up dieting. This program is all about rediscovering your natural appetite. If you are eating clean, healthy food, your natural appetite will determine for you how much to eat. If you eat dairyless, meatless, sugar-free, and chemical-free foods in the right combination, you will automatically or instinctually eat the right amount. In other words, eating this way means you really can "eat anything you want," because eventually the more you eat this kind of food, the more you will *want* this kind of food and this kind of food only. I can't tell you the number of times I have heard from people that once they cleansed their palate and could appreciate the healthy flavors of real food, they fell in love with the program and their excess weight came off. Portion control became a natural process. Everything in these recipes is good for you, good tasting, and will promote your body's function as a well-oiled machine. When you let your body do what it was designed to do, your metabolism—the burning of your food (storing of the good stuff and elimination of the waste)—happens naturally.

Of all the books I've written (five so far), this book has definitely been the most fun and tastiest to work on. I've learned so much from you through your E-mails and messages on my website, marilu.com, your comments at book signings, and talking to you on the street. I know that most of you want to eat tastier, healthier food made from ingredients that you already have or can find easily. That is why the recipes in this book are so easy and delicious. While many of them have come from restaurants and cookbooks, some of the best recipes in this book have come from readers like you. This book, inspired by you, contributed to by you, is, most importantly, for you. So come on. Let's have some fun in the kitchen!

Why You Should Cook for Yourself and Your Family

1. It's cheaper.
2. You will be using fresher food, thereby eating foods when vitamins, minerals, and flavors are at their peak.
3. You know what you're eating.
4. You're in control.
5. You won't get stuck with a lot of choices you don't want.
6. It's creative.
7. It's a way to share family time (get the kids involved!).
8. It's social.
9. It slows down the whole wonderful experience of eating. You enjoy the process rather than the goal-oriented approach to filling your gut.
10. You will have an investment in what you've made.
11. Like everything else, the more you do it, the better you become at it.
12. It can be fun.
13. If you bring home takeout, you tend to eat it so much faster.
14. No one would ever eat standing up after making a wonderful meal.
15. You will conquer your fear of being a cooking failure.

I Feel Better When:

1. I have energy.
2. I feel balanced.
3. I feel prepared.
4. I do my homework.
5. I can find something.
6. I've crossed something off my "to do" list.

7. I exercise every day or at least three times a week.
8. I drink one to two liters of water a day (between meals, of course).
9. I take time for myself.
10. I'm near my fighting weight (like a boxer!).
11. I've gotten a good night's sleep.
12. I listen to my body.
13. I do something for someone else.
14. I know my family is eating well.

1
Kitchen 101

Evaluating Your Kitchen

Depending on how organized, or disorganized, your kitchen is right now, a project like this can, at first, seem overwhelming. There is usually so much to do and it's hard to know where to begin or in what order you should attack the problem. Approach the process of detoxing your kitchen the same as you would detoxing your body—one step at a time. I'm sure that some of you have kitchens that already function like a Swiss watch. You guys can skip this chapter. But, for the rest of you (especially if your most important kitchen appliance is the telephone), carefully read on.

Before We Even Talk About Food, Let's See How Your Kitchen Functions

Think of this as Kitchen 101. Some of what I am going to say is so basic, you won't believe I'm explaining it. But as with any other 101 course, it's best to start at the beginning with the most fundamental explanations and principles. I have found that the best approach for every kitchen makeover is to use a simple and specific step-by-step process. So let's get started!

Step One   First and foremost, think about what it is you want to accomplish by organizing your kitchen. Set your goals and envision your kitchen's future layout and how you would like it to function. You may find it useful to make a list of all the things you would like your kitchen to be. Write down everything that you *don't* want it to be as well. You can keep a small kitchen makeover notebook and add to it as you go along. For example, some of the following statements may reflect the goals you have for your kitchen:

1. I want to make the most of my available kitchen space.
2. I always want to be able to find the specific utensil, knife, dish, pot, oven mitt, or appliance I need.
3. I want my spices and oils to be organized and within easy reach.
4. I want to be able to find in my refrigerator, freezer, and pantry what I want when I want it.
5. I don't want to waste food by allowing it to rot in my refrigerator or cupboards because I bought too much, bought the wrong item, or couldn't find it while it was buried somewhere in the back.
6. I don't want to ruin frozen food by allowing it to stay in the freezer so long that it becomes a victim of freezer burn.
7. I want the cleanup procedure after every meal to be fast, easy, and certainly not something I dread, put off until later, or have to beg others to help me with because it's so burdensome.
8. I don't want to have to worry about chemicals in the cleaning products under my sink being potentially dangerous for my children or for the rest of my family.

In this list, you may also want to include dietary goals for yourself and your family as well. For example:

1. I want to be able to prepare fresh, natural, healthy, vibrant, and tasty meals every day, or nearly every day.
2. I want the food I choose to give my family energy and to make us feel good rather than making us feel tired and not our best.
3. I want to limit my family's dependence on fast food, takeout, and/or unhealthy, unnatural, overprocessed food products.

This is just a sample list to help you get started. Now it's your turn. Feel free to write down all your thoughts and goals for your new kitchen. Writing it down doesn't obligate you to fulfill each and every wish. It's simply a good way for you to identify what you want to accomplish most, so don't hold back. Writing it down is the first step toward achieving your goal.

Step Two   Now that you've finished your kitchen wish list, analyze all the things you do now to prepare meals, or to *avoid* preparing meals. As in any makeover, what *doesn't* work is obvious. So let's start there. When I put this question to a group of moms, they came up with the following statements. See if you recognize your kitchen complaints in this list.

What's *Not* Working?

1. My kitchen is so disorganized I feel defeated before I even start.
2. My kitchen has no system. Dishes and silverware are scattered about and I can never find anything because nothing has a specific place.
3. I don't have enough counter space to do any convenient preparation of food.
4. My oven is so small I can't do any real cooking or baking.
5. I have no storage space in my cupboards to keep staples on hand, much less any specialty items.
6. My kitchen is incomplete. I don't know what pots or pans or utensils to buy to fill in the gaps.

7. I do other things in my kitchen. It's become my office. Everything gets dumped there, especially after shopping.
8. Nothing has a place, so everyone puts things back wherever they want.
9. Simple items like my paper towel dispenser need to be replaced, but I never think of it while I'm at the store.
10. I know I must childproof my cupboards and under the sink, but I haven't gotten around to it yet.
11. I don't know how to clean up after each step of preparation—as a result the end cleanup job is mountainous.
12. I often throw out leftovers because I can never find the right lid for my plastic containers.
13. The garbage tends to pile up because the garbage bags are hard to reach under the sink. Everybody puts off changing the bag because they hope somebody else will do it.
14. I don't have the right garbage can for the size of my kitchen or the amount of my garbage.
15. I have never figured out a garbage system that works well for the combination of wet and dry garbage that passes through my kitchen.

These are very common problems, so if they sound familiar, you're not alone. Make your list as lengthy as necessary.

Step Three Look through the recipe section in this book and pick out at least five recipes that you may want to prepare on a regular basis, and pick out another five that you might want to try for a special occasion. As you look over these recipes, be aware of what your kitchen is missing and what it would take in order to prepare these recipes efficiently. For example, if you were to choose a wide variety of dishes that you have never cooked before, you might need the following:

- a good chef's knife
- a good paring knife
- measuring cups and spoons
- a colander
- a large cutting board
- a steamer

- a loaf pan
- a baking dish
- wooden spoons
- infused olive oils
- fresh and dried basic spices (oregano, parsley, basil, rosemary, cumin)

After finishing these first three steps, you should now have an overall idea of what your kitchen is going to need. You don't have to buy anything yet. This is to help you envision your future kitchen's efficiency. You should refer back to your lists periodically to stay focused on your overall plan. Remember that you can always add to these lists as your needs or ideas change. You are now ready to take action.

Step Four Eliminate all unnecessary items from your kitchen. This includes expired foods, junk foods that you're ready to give up, things that belong somewhere else in your house, and so on. This is just the first pass. You'll be doing another elimination round of things that don't belong in your kitchen in Chapter 2, when we talk in detail about the dangerous chemicals in our food and household products. But this first pass is necessary to free up some space and help you get started. Work clockwise around your kitchen, starting with the refrigerator, since that's the core. It's important to stick with a specific and systematic order so that you can easily keep track of what you've done and haven't done.

As you move along, keep two items beside you, a garbage can and a cardboard box. On this first pass, focus on the items that are obvious. Throw into the garbage can *everything* that is garbage: expired and rotten food, old spices, foods that you know are unhealthy and you are ready to dump, and anything you haven't used or eaten in the last year or so. In the cardboard box, place all the things that you want to keep but need to move to another part of the house: clothes, tools, kids' artwork that is falling apart, et cetera. I am always amused by the things I find while doing kitchen makeovers: lingerie, tennis rackets, bowling trophies, dumbbells, wigs, you name it. One family even had their dead parakeet in their freezer for seven years!

The kitchen should be reserved for food and things connected with food. It is the most important room in the house. Make sure yours works at full capacity. Don't compromise your health because your kitchen is the catch-all. Once you have thrown out the garbage and/or returned the various items to the other parts of your home, you should have some newly available space in your kitchen so you can begin reorganizing it.

Step Five   Establish a specific and effective place for each item. This step requires some thought and creativity. There are two Golden Rules for organization and efficiency that must be followed.

1. Every item must have its own specific place. Choose one place and one place only for each item.
2. It's equally important that every item gets returned to its specific spot immediately after it has been used and/or cleaned.

This may sound overly meticulous, but if these two sacred rules are not followed, things will eventually get misused, misplaced, or lost forever. You'll be forced to buy a particular item again, and that one will eventually get lost, too. Then you'll have two of the same thing (somewhere!) and won't be using either one. (If, for example, you open a drawer and find a few pieces of silverware, coffee filters, and some birthday candles, chances are your utensil drawers need to be rethought.) It's important that your family understands what you're trying to accomplish. I have found, however, that if a place for an item makes sense, other family members will return the item to that same spot.

Here are a couple of suggestions to keep in mind as you design your newly organized kitchen:

1. Organize by category, so you'll always know where to find everything (e.g., dishes, silverware, plasticware, kids' items, and so on).
2. Place frequently used items within easy reach.
3. Place some items that are used in tandem close to each other (e.g., the cutting knives near the cutting board).
4. Establish a place for your utensils so they can be found (i.e., keep smaller utensils like potato peelers, can openers, etc., in their own space, separate from larger ones).
5. Know the size of your oven so that you will buy whole fish or poultry that will fit. (There's nothing worse than bringing home an eighteen-pound turkey for a fourteen-pound oven.)

6. Size up the shape of your fridge. Know its dimensions so that you don't overbuy. You may have to remove shelves or compartments to better organize your groceries.

It's a good idea to work in the same clockwise fashion that you did while you were removing the bad-guy items. So let's start with the refrigerator. Many people simply organize by putting the frozen foods in the freezer and the "refrigerate after opening" stuff in the rest of the fridge in whatever order they were opened. But some foods often get hidden in the back because they're shorter than the rest of their food friends. They get overlooked and eventually passed up for other less tasty, taller foods; and they die. It's a very sad story. (We lost our family tangerine this way.) Don't let this happen to you; instead, put taller foods in the back and group similar items together. It's also a good idea to keep fruits and vegetables in their own section, and check on them frequently (especially the tangerines!).

Shortage of space often forces people to put things wherever they can just to get them in there. To avoid this, I always do a quick inventory check before I go to the store. That way I rarely buy things I already have, and I get rid of the foods that are expired or containers that are now empty, or nearly empty. I've got three guys at home, ages four and a half, six, and fifty-two. All three of them know how to operate a computer, but none of them knows how to throw out an empty carton. They are pros at avoiding the responsibility by leaving everything one swig, bite, or piece away from being empty.

Now let's move on to the cupboard. Group similar items together (cans with cans, snack foods in a certain section). Again, it's best if you place taller foods in the back. Think of it as though you're a photographer and you're taking a class portrait. You can even designate your oatmeal as the class teacher. I like to think of my wild rice as the class clown. (You can't imagine how often I have to separate him from the kasha.) It may be a good idea to keep your packaged goods like pasta and cereal in plastic containers for easy reference and to keep them fresh and free from bugs. Remember to do inventory in the cupboard before shopping, too. All of this gets really easy once you establish it as a routine. These are just suggestions. The most important point to keep in mind is the way *you* would like to organize your kitchen and cook. And remember, just like your Total Health Makeover, this is a work in progress. You should be open to reevaluating and changing your kitchen system, as needed, in the future.

Try hanging a small dry-erase board on your kitchen wall. Make sure it has a marker attached that's always ready to spring into action. Use this to jot down thoughts, ideas, needed items, phone numbers, or anything that is not working in your kitchen procedure that needs to be changed. In my home, we use a large kitchen calendar on the wall to keep everyone's appointments straight, and a kitchen notebook on the counter to keep a grocery list. By making these sources available at all times, each member of the family feels like he or she can contribute to a well-run household and kitchen.

Creating an Efficient Dishwashing System

When I was growing up, my family's idea of an efficient dishwashing system was my sister Christal and I. She was responsible on Mondays, Wednesdays, Fridays, and Sunday afternoons. And I had Tuesday, Thursday, Saturday, and the dreaded Sunday night dinner. We had no dishwasher, of course, so the job for one little girl to clean the kitchen and wash and dry the entire dish load for eight people was daunting to say the least. But I learned to really appreciate and even enjoy my job. First of all, I liked the idea that dishwashing has a very definite beginning, middle, and end, unlike most tasks. And I really liked the fact that I could get better at my job if I could figure out more efficient ways of getting the job done. I learned strategies for doing an unappealing task in the most appealing ways possible. And here are some of these principles I use to this day.

1. Take pride in your job and believe in your heart that you're the only one who can do it really well.
2. Break down the job into a series of steps, and as you complete each one, cross it off the imaginary list in your head.
3. Try to accomplish another task while doing the task at hand. For example, while I was washing dishes I would try to sing the entire score of a Broadway musical. I would size up the load to determine what show would get the job done. I would keep singing until the kitchen sparkled and I could take my bow.

Perhaps the idea of singing your way to a clean kitchen doesn't appeal to you, but nevertheless, the importance of an efficient dishwashing system is obvious. If your pots, pans, and dishes are dirty and out of commission, your whole system shuts down. That's why it's essential that your dishwashing system be fast and efficient. Let's face it. Washing dishes is not really fun. We prefer to spend as little time doing it as necessary. The best way to save time is to get to it as soon as possible. I know it's nice to sit and relax after dinner, but the sooner you rinse and soak that dish, the less overall effort will be required to get it cleaned, dried, and put away.

Besides, you can have it both ways. Hang out with company, but make sure you have hot, soapy water waiting for your dishes as you clear the table. I've always found that once you get your dishes soaking, you're more than halfway there. Get the soapy water ready before you even start preparing the meal, so you can rinse, soak, or even wash each knife, shredder, or bowl immediately after you finish using it. This is also an important step for water conservation. Imagine how much more water is required to clean something after the food has already hardened. If your soaking procedure is not working well right now, perhaps your space is limited or your dishpan is too small. Whatever the problem, figure it out, and correct it.

If you have a dishwasher, the same rule applies (rinse ASAP). With commercial dishwashers, I've found that less detergent is needed than what the manufacturer recommends. Try using about half or two-thirds of what you would normally use. Remember that fine knives, wooden spoons, and pots with wooden handles must *always* be washed (and dried!) by hand. It's rewarding to always have your dishes cleaned and organized. In fact, make it a point to start your meal preparation with an empty dishwasher. There's nothing worse than a sink full of dirty dishes waiting to be loaded and a dishwasher full of dishes waiting to be cleaned. Dirty dishes create a lot of subconscious stress for people, not to mention the potential health hazard that comes from letting them pile up.

Creating an Efficient Garbage System

If you read the chapter called "What's the Poop" in my book *The Total Health Makeover*, you know how important I believe bowel function is for overall health. I will spare you the funky details for *this* book, but I bring it up because I feel that the garbage system in a home is the key to efficient organization just as bowel function is the key to overall body function. It's all about taking out the trash, and when either one gets backed up, you've got trouble! *Never* let your garbage get backed up, especially in the kitchen! When I shared a studio apartment in New York with a former boyfriend, his one and only household responsibility was taking out the garbage. All this involved was dropping it down the incinerator right outside our door. He always let it pile up so high, I eventually gave in and threw it out myself. One day, I completely lost it and screamed at him while he was in the shower. He angrily bolted out of the bathroom and said, "You want me to throw out the garbage? Fine! I'll throw out the garbage!"

He grabbed all eleven bags in one scoop and charged out in the hallway buck naked. I quickly shut the door behind him and locked it. The next thing I heard was a quiet voice saying, "Mar? Come on. Open the door. This isn't funny."

Then I heard him say timidly to our neighbor, "Hi, Mr. Razen . . . er . . . my girlfriend's a real comedienne."

I finally let him in. He was so angry, but it was totally worth it!

The moral of the story is this: If you're going to throw out the garbage in your birthday suit, at least save something for your protection: a Twinkie wrapper, a banana peel, or in my boyfriend's case, the Sunday *New York Times*! (He wasn't all bad!) Throwing out garbage should never feel like a chore. It should always be something you do without thought or obstacles. If you can't immediately find a place to throw something out, you may put it off until later and it will accumulate. The best way to avoid this is to establish a smooth and smart system. Here are a few suggestions:

1. Buy garbage bags in bulk. You'll save money and never put off changing a bag because you don't have a fresh replacement waiting in the wings.
2. Avoid cheap brands. They may seem like a bargain, but the headaches aren't worth it. Nothing is worse than a broken bag of leaky garbage.
3. Make sure every room in your house has at least one garbage container; some rooms may need two. I recommend investing in a really good container for the kitchen. Take your time shopping; it's worth the effort. If you hate odors, get one with a lid. Consider the kind you have to step on to raise the top, especially if you're phobic about touching the lid.
4. Save paper bags for newspapers and plastic bags for plastic and glass bottle recycling.

Whatever garbage system you design, try to keep the environmental three *R*s in mind: Reduce, Reuse, and Recycle.

2

Out with the
Bad Stuff!

You have already done one pass of throwing out surface garbage. Now let's focus on a different kind of garbage: meat, sugar, dairy, and chemicals. It is the kind most Americans eat, ingest, inhale, and touch every day. If you are familiar with the "rules of the road" from *The Total Health Makeover* and *The 30-Day Total Health Makeover* and understand why I don't recommend you eat meat, dairy, and sugar, you can skip the next few paragraphs. However, if you have never read any of my books before, or need to be reminded, please read on.

Getting Rid of the Health Robbers
in Your Refrigerator, Freezer, and Pantry

Meat

Meat eaters, especially red-meat eaters, are three times as likely as vegetarians to suffer from heart disease and breast cancer. Meat eating stresses the liver and kidneys, two important detoxifying organs. It can also deplete calcium, which adds to the risk of osteoporosis, and the uric acid in meat can deposit in our joints, inflaming arthritis.

People who eat red meat five or more times a week increase their risk for colon cancer by 400 percent compared to people who eat no meat or eat it less than once a month. Women who eat beef, lamb, or pork as a daily staple are two and a half times more likely to develop colon cancer than women who eat meat less than once a month. The substitution of other protein sources such as beans and lentils is known to reduce the risk of colon cancer. Prostate cancer is another risk. Meats are higher in animal fat, which is harder for us to digest and therefore stays in our bodies longer.

Humans were meant to be primarily vegetarian. Our closest living relatives from the animal world, apes, are vegetarians. Even cows are, by nature, vegetarians. The structure of our skin, teeth, stomach, and bowels, and the length of our digestive system, are all typically vegetarian. Somewhere along the way, we overcame our physical limitations and decided to kill other animals for food. Unfortunately, we've become too smart for our own good. Please leave meat for the carnivores. Contrary to what many people believe, we are not carnivores. Our incisors (canine teeth) are not long enough or sharp enough, and our digestive tract is not designed to efficiently process meat.

We can survive quite easily on a diet that consists of no animal products, a vegan diet. Most of the world's human population is, for the most part, vegetarian. All of the negative information claiming that vegetarian diets lack some necessary nutrients and protein comes from organizations, such as the Meat and Livestock Commission, that compete with vegetable food sources for their profits.

Also, I often hear people say, "I don't feel strong when I don't eat meat. Meat gives me strength." Well . . . the largest and strongest dinosaurs were vegetarians. Elephants, who are big, strong, *and* smart, are vegetarians. Eating meat has nothing to do with strength. In fact, it zaps your strength because it overtaxes your digestive system and wears you out. A chimpanzee is 97 percent vegetarian. Orangutans are more than 99 percent vegetarian. Both are extremely close in DNA to humans. Chimpanzees are much closer to us than they are to any other animal, and they eat a much healthier diet than we do. (Are we *sure* we're smarter?)

Even if humans were built like carnivores (and we're definitely not), we would still have to contend with the added hormones, antibiotics, tranquilizers, additives, preservatives, and pesticides found in most meat sources today.

People often ask me whether or not I eat chicken. When I first started this program, I didn't plan to give up chicken. But about two and a half years after I gave up red meat, chicken began to taste funny to me. I became more aware that its texture and density made it too hard for me to digest, and its smell and taste no longer appealed to me. So I gave it up. At that time "free-range" chicken products were not widely available. Today, I still don't eat chicken, and I don't really recommend it in the long run for women because I believe it is too concentrated a protein for females. My husband and sons eat a little chicken as long as it is free range. It's important that chicken is free range because then the chicken is raised on natural grains and allowed to run free as opposed to being shot up with steroids and growth hormones and cooped up in tiny cages. (You don't want to inherit all the chemicals and "stress" that come with a conventional chicken.)

Sugar

In recent years, sugar has been blamed for conditions such as hyperactivity, diabetes, hypoglycemia, bad moods, yeast infections, obesity, and tooth decay. Sugar depletes your body of all of the B vitamins. It leaches calcium from your hair, blood, bones, and teeth. It interferes with the absorption of calcium, protein, and other minerals in your body and retards the growth of valuable intestinal bacteria. This is what we often give to our valentines. How sweet!

Sugar has a fermenting effect in your stomach. It stops the secretion of gastric juices and inhibits the stomach's ability to digest. People eat desserts at the end of their meals because it makes them feel emotionally satisfied. But because sugar inhibits the stomach's ability to digest, it makes the food that accompanies the sugar stagnate, making it more fattening. It's not the fat or calories in sugar that's a problem. It's what sugar does to your digestive enzymes. That's the problem. Sugar is not digested in the mouth like other foods. When eaten alone, it passes directly into the small intestine, but when eaten with other foods, it gets stuck in the stomach for a while. Sugar in the stomach is a sure way to guarantee rapid acid fermentation in the warm and moist conditions that exist there. So, drinking a regular soda with your meal or sugar in your coffee while eating breakfast definitely ignites that fire. It's like you've got a winery working inside your stomach.

Kicking the sugar habit isn't an easy thing to do. I know when I decided to give up sugar, it was very difficult for me. My theory on this one is that once you start eating sugar, you want more and more of it, even if your stomach tells you it's full. That is what I call the sugar treadmill. It goes beyond satisfying a simple urge. People generally eat to fill their stomachs, not caring what they put into it. But you *should* care, because so much of how we feel and think and act is all tied to what we eat, right?

Getting caught up on a sugar treadmill is dangerous, especially for children. I have often referred to sugar as "kiddy cocaine," because, in my opinion, that is exactly what it is. Watching your children's behavior change right before your very eyes after they've eaten sugar can be a very dramatic experience. It is like giving the child a drug. It stimulates, causes mood swings, and can be addicting. (Sounds like a drug to me!) Giving your child sugar is such an unhealthy food choice (if you want to call it a food). It only stimulates and trains him or her to behave in an unruly and unhealthy way.

Americans consume somewhere in the neighborhood of 136 pounds of sugar per person, per year. Sugar adds "empty" (meaning of no nutritional value) calories to your daily intake. Over half of the sugar consumed today is added directly from the sugar bowl while eating or preparing a meal. The food manufacturers add the other half, either as sugar or as high-fructose corn syrup. Your body breaks down sugar that you eat into the sugar found in the blood, called glucose.

If you want to get off that sugar treadmill, pick one of two ways: either cut down on your total sugar intake by eliminating added sugars and slowly decreasing your intake of foods that are high in sugar, or go cold turkey. Give up all added sugar and any food that has refined white sugar in it. It's that simple.

I found when I gave up white sugar, I also ended up giving up red meat. They are total opposites in terms of being yin (sugar) and yang (meat). The reason you crave one with the other is that they balance each other out because they're both so extreme in the food spectrum. It's hard to eat one without the other, just as it's hard to entirely give up one and still crave the other. Dropping both from your diet makes it easier to stick with not eating either food, because your craving for both goes way down. The more vegetable protein you eat in place of animal protein, the lower your desire for sugar will be. You'll see! That craving for something sweet at the end of a meal slowly fades because now you're eating a much more balanced meal.

Once you decide to kick the sugar habit, you'll notice that your taste buds will start picking up flavors and sensations you may have never experienced before. Everything you eat will start to taste better and be more alive with flavor. Oddly enough, it's not the food that tastes better; it's your body that's now able to taste the food better. (You'll find that this is a common and wonderful little dividend that comes from improving your diet.)

Dairy

I have been virtually dairy free since 1979. Believe me when I tell you quite frankly that eliminating dairy from your diet will change your life forever. It'll change the way you look and feel and add years to your life. When I first talk to people about this program, they invariably say to me, "There is no way I could ever give up milk or cheese." The overwhelming response is that they might be able to deal with all of the other aspects of this health makeover, but the dairy thing, well, that just seems downright impossible! I should know. When a nutritionist first suggested that I give up dairy, I was one of those people! But after reading about the connection between dairy and heart disease, and arthritis, and diabetes, and kidney stones, and allergies, and nasal congestion, and depression, and respiratory problems, I thought, "Wowww! I owe it to myself to try this."

Once I finally got off dairy for good, my face changed so much. My perpetual puffiness was finally gone. That baby fat layer, brought on and maintained because of my dairy consumption, went away. I actually had bone structure! My resemblance to Miss Piggy was a thing of the past. My lungs and kidneys were functioning better because they were no longer clogged by the dairy sludge that had been impairing their function.

Everyone who goes off dairy raves about having more energy, better digestion, and feeling less stuffy in their nose. I can't think of anyone who didn't feel a difference once they gave up dairy. Some, unfortunately, go back to eating some dairy, but they never go back to the amount they consumed before. They now know consciously that they shouldn't be eating dairy.

I'm always saying that the only thing milk is designed to do is to turn a fifty-pound calf into a three-hundred-pound cow in six months. If cows don't drink milk, why should we? Think of how strange it would be to drink something like orangutan's milk? Yet it would make more sense for us to drink orangutan milk because we are closer to them as a species than we are to cows.

Humans were never meant to consume anything other than human breast milk, and that *only* while we're infants. We are the only animals that drink the milk of another animal. Milk is a food of convenience, and in our quest for convenience, we have made ourselves one of the sickest animals on the face of the earth. This is another example of man being too smart for his own good. In many countries, the thought of drinking milk from a cow is as absurd as drinking milk from an orangutan. Milk is nature's food for a baby calf, which has four stomachs and will double its weight in forty-seven days. Not only does a baby calf have four stomachs, it also has nine feet of intestines, as opposed to humans, who have twenty-seven feet of intestines. Our digestive enzymes are not capable of breaking down a food that is designed to nurse the young of another species. Our stomachs don't even recognize dairy as a "food," and everything we eat with it becomes difficult to digest.

Maybe you're thinking to yourself, "What about all of the good things we hear about milk, like it helps build calcium and keeps our bones strong?" Although millions of dollars are spent every year photographing celebrities with white mustaches proclaiming the virtues of milk, the truth is that the calcium in cow's milk is much coarser than in human milk, and the human body does not adequately absorb it. Also, all of the processing of dairy products reduces the calcium supply in those products, so it becomes very difficult to use pasteurized, homogenized, or other processed dairy products as a good source of calcium. In fact, most of us get enough calcium through other foods we eat, so we don't need to get it from milk. Spinach, broccoli, and all other green leafy vegetables contain calcium. Soybeans, tofu, nuts, and sesame seeds are also excellent sources of calcium. So are salmon and sardines. Even concentrated fruits like dates, figs, and prunes offer up enough calcium for your body's needs. Cows get their calcium from eating grass in the fields where they graze. (You don't really think they're getting their calcium from eating a pizza, do you?) Next time you go to drink a glass of milk, think of it as cow breast milk. Or better yet (my favorite phrase for it) . . . bovine slime. In fact, my slogan on my last book tour was "Get rid of bovine slime, get rid of bovine butt." Wake up, America. "Got Milk?" Well, I say, "Not Milk!"

Butter

Making butter requires 21.2 pounds of milk for each "finished" pound of butter. One quart of milk weighs 2.15 pounds. The fat found in dairy products is animal fat, which is high in cholesterol. Whole milk and anything made from whole milk is very high in saturated fat, which can increase your cholesterol level. *Saturated* is a chemical term that means the fat molecule is completely covered with hydrogen atoms. Without those atoms, the fat is *unsaturated*. Saturated fats stimulate your liver to make more cholesterol. Most animal products contain substantial amounts of saturated fat. Lose dairy, and you'll lose fat.

Now that you've heard all of this about meat, sugar, and dairy, it's time to go through your kitchen once again for a second pass. Start again with your refrigerator and work clockwise. This time keep the following information handy to help motivate you and help you decide what to keep and what to dump. You can even photocopy it out of the book and tape it to your refrigerator.

MEAT

- People who eat red meat five or more times a week are three times as likely to suffer from heart disease and breast cancer, and four times as likely to develop colon cancer than people who eat no meat or eat it less than once a month.
- Meat overtaxes the digestive system, stresses the liver and kidneys, depletes calcium, and deposits uric acid in our joints.
- The structure of our skin, teeth, stomach, bowels, and length of our digestive system are all typical of vegetarian animals.
- Our closest relatives in the animal kingdom, chimps, are 97 percent vegetarian.
- 90 percent of the pesticides Americans consume comes not from vegetables and fruit, as most people assume, but from meat and dairy products.
- Animal products are the number one cause of our number one killer, heart disease. It kills more people in the United States each year than the *combined* total of U.S. combat deaths in WWI, WWII, Vietnam, and Korea.

SUGAR

- Depletes the body of B vitamins.
- Leaches calcium from hair, blood, bones, and teeth.
- Interferes with the absorption of calcium, protein, and other minerals.
- Retards growth of valuable intestinal bacteria.
- Overstimulates and causes dramatic mood swings in children, making them unruly. (I call it "kiddy cocaine.")
- Research has connected it with diabetes, obesity, rheumatism, gout, hypoglycemia, acne, indigestion, arteriolosclerosis, and even mental illness.
- Ferments in the stomach, stops the secretion of gastric juices, and inhibits the stomach's ability to digest.
- Forget what Mary Poppins says. A spoonful is not a harmless aid for getting the medicine down. In fact, you'll need medicine if you get too much of it down.

DAIRY

- In studies, has been linked to heart disease, arthritis, childhood diabetes, kidney stones, allergies, nasal congestion, depression and mood swings, respiratory problems, canker sores, and mad cow disease.
- A high percentage of cow's milk contains bovine growth hormones that are unnatural and unhealthy for humans.
- It's a myth that milk and dairy products are a necessary source of calcium.
- Cow's milk is designed to turn a 50-pound baby calf into a 300-pound young cow, and that's it! If you don't have aspirations like that, don't drink it!

Additives and Preservatives

You might be saying to yourself, "I don't really have to worry that much about food chemicals and additives; after all, we've got the FDA, the USDA, the EPA, the CDC, and even the FBI looking out for us. All those guys from agencies with big letters go to work every day to test and retest everything to make sure we won't ever harm or poison ourselves. These additives wouldn't be legal if they weren't okay to eat. Right?"

WRONG!!! As well-intentioned as those big government agencies are, the job of determining whether everything is safe is beyond overwhelming! It's actually impossible. There are over three thousand chemical additives being used in our foods today. The FDA cannot even be sure how dangerous the few additives that have been tested are, much less the majority that have been barely looked at. Testing is very complicated. It takes twenty to thirty years for the dangers of some chemicals to reveal themselves. Often additives that originally got the green light are later found to be dangerous. Most of these chemicals are not naturally found in nature, have never been seen before, and are often combined in new ways with other new substances. Most additives have not been tested alone, much less in a synergistic combination.

These government agencies are understaffed and underfinanced, and sometimes lack the sophisticated technology required to handle this unbelievably complex job. (There *is* a price to pay for lower taxes.) Ultimately, the job to protect yourself and your family is *yours*. Here's what we currently face:

- The GRAS (Generally Regarded as Safe) rating by the FDA is determined by the manufacturers, not by the FDA. (That's like allowing high school students to grade themselves.)
- Some additives are allowed because they cause severe allergic reactions only in *some* people. At present, it's up to you, not the government, to determine if you're one of those allergic people.
- 80 percent of U. S. livestock and poultry are treated with drugs.
- Almost one hundred different pesticides are currently being used to control insect infestation of our crops and our livestock. Many of these pesticides are already known to cause cancer.
- Because of the ever-increasing use of antibiotics on our animals, strains of bacteria have become stronger and much more resistant to antibiotics.

- We must learn to read between the lines of food labels, since manufacturers are allowed to make misleading and false claims like ALL NATURAL INGREDIENTS or ALL NATURAL FLAVORS.

As bad as this sounds, I believe that our government is trying to move in the right direction. Unfortunately, powerful interest groups often hold them back. The food pyramid introduced in 1992 is a good example of this. Fats, oils, meats, and dairy got the highest positions on the pyramid, helping consumers overlook the fact that those sections are, in actuality, the smallest and *least* recommended. Originally it was supposed to be a pie chart, not a pyramid. But the meat and dairy lobbyists won the battle and got their misleading food pyramid. They feared a pie chart would present too clear a picture and increase public health awareness (their biggest fear of all).

The government has, however, been tougher on food producers recently, tightening their regulations on food labels. Over the next twenty years, they're hoping to lower national health care costs by forcing the food producers to use more honest labeling. The government believes that better labeling will force producers to make healthier products, and people will become wiser consumers and make healthier choices. It's our responsibility, right now, to learn as much as we can about what *is* actually known and to carefully read between the lines of every label of each product we buy.

Commonly Used Additives

The following is a discussion and listing of the most commonly used additives. I hope this will help you decide what you should keep and what you should immediately throw away.

As I stated earlier, there are over three thousand additives currently being used. Categorizing them in some sort of best-to-worst fashion would not only be exhausting, it would be impossible. There are far too many variables in many cases to say which is better or worse for our health; however, we can, in a general way, categorize them into three basic groups. Some additives are obviously dangerous, some are probably okay, and then there is a middle category that is not so easily defined. This is at least a start that is necessary so that we can begin to identify the additives that pose the most serious health risks.

Category 1   *Commonly used additives you should avoid completely because of one or more of the following reasons*

- Were found to be carcinogenic (cancer causing)
- Caused tumors and/or other serious side effects in lab animals
- Contribute to heart, lung, or kidney disease
- Are connected with birth defects
- Are associated with nausea or vomiting
- Contain a potentially dangerous level of toxicity
- Were given a GRAS (Generally Recognized as Safe) rating by the FDA *but* have also been associated with dangerous health risks

Approval for the GRAS rating is determined by the additive manufacturers themselves and not by the FDA as it once was. The procedure was recently changed in order to save time and paperwork. The manufacturers, however, are required to show some evidence to support their GRAS status, and this helps promote an openness regarding their products. The result of this is that the GRAS list really doesn't mean much at all. For the most part, though, most of the truly dangerous additives don't have a GRAS rating and most of the safer additives do. (But keep in mind that many former GRAS members are now considered to be harmful by the government.)

Category 2 *Additives that have risk factors that are unclear for any of the following reasons*

- May cause an allergic reaction in *some* people, but not everyone
- Are not sufficiently tested yet
- Cause side effects that are relatively minor
- Cause serious side effects but only from abnormally large doses

Category 3 *Additives that are probably okay and might even be good for us for the following reason*

- Found to be harmless and/or contain some nutritional value (as opposed to some additives that have nutritional value but don't make it in this category because they also have negative aspects)

Note: I use the word *probably* with caution, since history has taught us that many additives that were found to be "okay" at one particular time turned out to be dangerous a few years later.

If you listen to your body and eliminate meat, sugar, dairy, and all the foods that contain additives found in Category 1, you should consider that a very good start on the road to good health.

KEY

A   Probably carcinogenic (cancer causing)

B   Caused serious side effects in lab animals

C   May contribute to heart or lung disease

D   May contribute to gastrointestinal, liver, or kidney disease

E   May cause birth defects

F   Associated with nausea or vomiting

G   Toxic

H   Adversely affects the central nervous system

I   May adversely affect brain function and memory

J   May weaken the immune system

K   Causes common allergic reactions (runny nose, rash, etc.)

L   Not sufficiently tested

M   Relatively minor side effects

N   Serious side effects from abnormally large doses

P   Allergic reactions for some

GRAS   Generally regarded as safe by the FDA. (This doesn't necessarily mean it's safe. For example, cyclamates were once on this list. And, believe it or not, BHA, BHT, and MSG are still on it.)

CATEGORY ONE
(Most Dangerous)

Acesulfame-K: (A, B)

Acesulfame-potassium: (A, B)

Acetal: (C)

Acetaldehyde: (H) GRAS

Alkyl gallate: (D)

Alkyl sulfide: (C, D)

Aloe extract: (D)

Aluminum: (D, I, L)

Ammonium: (D)

Amyl acetate: (H)

Amyl alcohol: (G)

Animal or vegetable
    shortening: (C)

Artemisia: (D, H)

Artificial color FD&C: (A, H, I)

Aspartame: (E, H, I)

Aspergillus oryzae: (A)

Azo dyes: (C, D)

Benzyl alcohol: (F)

BHA: (A, B, D, E, J) GRAS

BHT: (A, B, D, E, J) GRAS

Biphenyl: (F)

Blue No. 1: (A, C, K, L)

Blue No. 2: (B, C, K)

Boric acid: (G)

Borneol: (D, H)

Brominated vegetable oil:
    (C, D, E)

Butylated hydroxyanisole-BHA:
    (A, B, D, E, J) GRAS

Butylated hydroxytoluene-BHT:
    (A, B, D, E, J) GRAS

Caffeine: addictive drug (C, D,
    E, H, I) GRAS

Calcium chloride: (C, D) GRAS

Calcium glucanate: (C, D) GRAS

Calcium lactate: (C, D) GRAS

Camphor oil: (E)

Caramel: (A) GRAS

Carboxymethylcellulose: (B)
    GRAS

Carrageenan: (A)

Carvacrol: (C, G)

Chlorine dioxide: (A)

Cinnamaldehyde: (D, K) GRAS

Coal tar dyes: (C, D, K)

Cocoa: Contains caffeine

Corn sugar: (C, D, H, M) GRAS

Corn syrup: (C, D, H, M)

Cyclamates: (A)

Dimethylpolysiloxane: (D)

Dioctyl sodium sulfosuccinate
    (DSS): (D, E, L)

Diphenyl: (F, K)

Disodium phosphate: (C, D)
    GRAS

EDTA: (D, K)

Equal: (E, H, I)—see
    Aspartame

Ethyl acetate: (D, H) GRAS

Ethyl methyl phenylglycidate: (B)

Ethyl vanillin: (B) GRAS

FD&C Blue No.1: (A, C, K, L)

FD&C Blue No.2: (B, C, K)

FD&C Citrus Red No. 2: (A)

FD&C Green No. 3: (A)

FD&C Red No. 3: (B)

FD&C Red No. 40: (H)

FD&C Yellow No. 5: (D, K)

FD&C Yellow No. 6: (A, B)

Formaldehyde: (A, E, G)

Free glutamates: (I)

Fructose: (C, D)

Glycerin: (F) GRAS

Heptylparaben: (E, L)

High fructose corn syrup: (C, D) GRAS

Hydrogen peroxide: (A) GRAS

Hydrogenated vegetable oil: (A, C)

Hydrolyzed vegetable protein: (H, I)

Imitation flavoring: (D, H)

Isolated soy protein: (F, I) if it contains nitrites

Leavening: May contain BHA and BHT.

Mannitol: (D, F, L)

MSG (monosodium glutamate): (E, D, H, I, K)

Nitrates: (A) Very dangerous carcinogen!

Nitrites: (A, F, I) Also very dangerous!

Olean and Olestra: (D)

Partially hydrogenated vegetable oil: (A, C)

Phenylmethyl cyclosiloxane: (B, D)

Phosphates: (D)

Polyxyethylene stearate: (D, K)

Potassium acetate: (D)

Potassium alginate: (C, D)

Potassium benzoate: (C, D, K) GRAS

Potassium bisulfite: (C,D)

Potassium bromate: (A, D, H)

Potassium chloride: (C, D, F) GRAS

Potassium nitrate: (A) a.k.a. nitrates

Potassium nitrite: (A, F, I) a.k.a. nitrites

Quinine: (E, L)

Saccharin: (A) Very dangerous!

Salatrim: (F, L)

Sodium acetate: (C, D)

Sodium alginate: (C, D, E)

Sodium aluminum sulfate: (B, I)

Sodium bisulfite: (C, G)

Sodium carbonate: (C, D)

Sodium nitrate: (A) a.k.a.
nitrates

Sodium nitrite: (A, F, I) a.k.a.
nitrites

Sodium polyphosphate: (D)

Vegetable shortening: (A, C)

Whey (dairy product): (C, D)

Whey protein concentrate
(dairy product): (C, D)

CATEGORY TWO
*Unclear (not sufficiently tested)
or associated with less serious
problems*

Acacia gum: (K,L) GRAS

Acetate: (N)

Acetic acid: (M) GRAS

Agar-agar: (N) GRAS

Alpha tocopherol acetate: (N)

Amylases: (P)

Angelica: (M) GRAS

Arabinogalactan: (L)

Ascorbic acid: (M) GRAS

Ascorbyl palmitate: (M) GRAS

Baking powder: may contain
aluminum

Barley malt: (M, P)

Benzaldehyde: (H, J, M)

Benzoate of soda: (D, K) GRAS

Benzoic acid: (D, K) GRAS

Benzyl acetate: (D)

Benzyl formate: (N)

Bergamot: (M)

Blackstrap molasses: (M)

Brown algae: (L) GRAS

Calcium phosphate: (D) GRAS

Calcium sulphate: (B) GRAS

Capsicum: (D) GRAS

Carmine: (L)

Carob bean gum: (L, P) GRAS

Casein: (P) GRAS

Castor oil: (N)

Citric acid: (M) GRAS

Clove bud oil: (M)

Clove leaf oil: (M)

Clover: (M)

Coconut oil: (C)

Corn gluten: (P) GRAS

Corn starch: (K, M) GRAS

Dill: (M) GRAS

Dill oil: (N)

Disodium guanylate: (L, M, P)

Disodium inosinate: (L, M, P)

Erythorbic acid: (K, P) GRAS

Ethyl alcohol: (C, N) GRAS fatal
in large doses

Formic acid: (M)

Fruit juice concentrate: (D, P)

Fumaric acid: (K, L, P) GRAS

Glucose: (M)

Gluten: (K, P)

Invert sugar: (M, P) GRAS

L-ascorbic acid: (D, N)

Licorice: (C, N) GRAS

Mace/nutmeg: (N) GRAS
very dangerous hallucino-
genic drug in high doses

Magnesium compounds:
(P) GRAS

Menadione: (M)

Modified food starch: (L) GRAS

Mono- and diglycerides: (C, D,
K, L) GRAS

Niacin: (M) GRAS

Nickel: (M, N) GRAS

Nitrous oxide: (B, M, P) GRAS

Paprika: (N) GRAS

Parabens: (L) GRAS

Pectins: (M) GRAS

Saffron: (N) GRAS

St. John's bread gum: (K, L)
GRAS

Salicylates: (P)

Salt: (C, D, P) GRAS

Silica: (D)

Sodium acetate: (C, D) GRAS

Sodium alginate: (C, D) GRAS

Sodium chloride: (C, D, P)
GRAS

Sodium sulfate: (C, D)

Stearic acid (may come from
hydrogenated oils): GRAS

Sucrose: (D, M) GRAS

Turmeric: (M) GRAS

Vegetable gum: (L)

Vitamin A: (N) GRAS

Vitamin A acetate: (N) GRAS

Vitamin A palmitate: (N) GRAS

Vitamin D2: (N) GRAS

Vitamin D3: (N) GRAS

Wheat gluten: (P) GRAS

Xanthan gum: (D, M)

Zinc chloride: (K, M) GRAS

Zinc sulfate: (B, D) GRAS

CATEGORY THREE:
*(Currently considered safe
and/or nutritional)**

Acetoin: GRAS

Acetyl methylcarbinol: GRAS

Aconitic acid: GRAS

Adiptic acid: GRAS

Alfalfa: GRAS

Allspice: GRAS

Annatto

Bakers yeast glycan

Bakers yeast protein

Beta-carotene: GRAS

Biotin: GRAS

Calcium glycerophosphate: GRAS

Calcium pyrophosphate: GRAS

Carbon dioxide: GRAS

Carotene: GRAS

Choline bitartrate: GRAS

Choline chloride: GRAS

Decanal: GRAS

Dillseed

Ergocalciferol

Ethyl butyrate: GRAS

Ethyl heptanoate: GRAS

Folcin

Folic acid

Fruit pectin

Garlic: GRAS

Ground limestone: GRAS

Inositol: GRAS

L-cysteine: GRAS

L-lysine

Lactoflavin

Lecithin: GRAS

Menaquinone

Nitrogen: GRAS

Pantothenic acid

Peptones: GRAS

Phytonadione

Quicklime: GRAS

Rennet: GRAS

Stevia

Taurine

Vitamin B_{12} GRAS

Wheat bran

Wheat germ

* WARNING! When looking over this third category of supposedly "safe" additives, keep in mind that most of them are nutrient additives that are often used to falsely add nutritional value to some of the most overrefined products of all. Therefore, the presence of some of these additives is frequently a sign that the food product is highly refined and probably contains additives from Category 1 as well. Also, the chemicals used to prepare these nutrients don't have to be listed on the label.

The best thing to keep in mind while you're shopping and reading labels is this: look for ingredients that sound like *real food*. Don't make yourself crazy, but stay away from labels that have a really long list of ingredients. That is almost always a sign of overprocessing and bad chemicals. And whatever you do, avoid any ingredients that would earn more than thirty-five points in Scrabble!

The Dangers of Aluminum, Teflon, and Stainless Steel in Pots and Pans

Aluminum and Teflon are cheaper than other types of cookware, which is why they're more popular. But I recommend that you eventually invest in one of the other more durable and safer options, such as porcelain enamel, cast iron, Corningware, glass, or stoneware. Both Teflon and aluminum dissolve easily into food. Teflon can enter food because it is so easily scratched, and aluminum leaches into food. Even when simple tap water is boiled, it becomes charged with aluminum. Many foods contain an abundance of acids and alkalies that dissolve aluminum. Avoid, especially, cooking highly acidic foods like tomatoes in aluminum. Cleansers and hard water will also dissolve aluminum. Studies link aluminum to cancer, migraines, severe intestinal disorders, and deterioration of the intellect.

Aluminum salts are another problem. Foods that are cooked in aluminum can react with it and form aluminum salts. These salts have been linked in many studies to mental, gastrointestinal, and cardiovascular disorders. Aluminum is, in fact, banned in several countries throughout the world. Buying it is not worth the savings. In fact, you'll save money in the long run if you invest in one of the safer options. Even if it weren't dangerous to your health, aluminum cookware is not very durable, and you can often taste it in your food. I don't recommend using aluminum foil, either, if you're wrapping something high in acidity like tomatoes or tomato-based sauces or pastas.

So what should you use? Well, unfortunately, not stainless steel; it might also be dangerous. Once it is scoured, tiny chromium and nickel particles, both very toxic, may be released from the stainless steel and leach into the food. The good news is that glass, cast iron, and porcelain-enamel-coated cast iron are still considered acceptable. These are all relatively easy to find, but, I'll admit, they're harder to find than aluminum, stainless steel, and Teflon. I'm not saying that you should throw out all of your pots and pans now, but you should eventually replace them with the safer alternatives.

If, after switching over, you really miss the old Teflon and its nonstick capabilities, try this little tip: heat the pan first, then add the oil, then add the food.

Harmful Chemicals Under Your Sink

Most of us are concerned about bacteria, germs, mold, mildew, and bugs in our homes, especially in our kitchens and bathrooms; however, the products containing harmful chemicals that we use to clean and disinfect are sometimes more dangerous than the biological contaminants we're trying to get rid of. This issue of harmful household chemicals is a complex one. Common household products can be dangerous to our health and to the health of our environment as well. We often assume that we're not in any danger as long as we don't get harmful products splashed in our eyes or swallow them. We also feel that everything is fine as long as we don't have any acute or chronic symptoms of chemical poisoning like headache, nausea, or severe allergies, so we feel there's no need to change any of our products or procedures.

Unfortunately, the harmful effects from long-term *secondary* exposure to toxic chemicals often go unnoticed until they become serious. Secondary exposure includes absorption through the skin and/or inhalation through the nose and mouth. We can absorb harmful chemicals through our skin in the same way that nicotine and other drug patch medications are delivered into the bloodstream. Even trace residues from a product applied to a table or countertop weeks ago could be hazardous to the touch. Long-term chronic poisoning like this can be as dangerous as the immediate acute poisoning that comes from swallowing, because we don't take immediate action. And it's not just the really toxic products with the bold and obvious skull-and-crossbone warning labels that are potentially dangerous. Even products as innocent-sounding as dishwashing liquid, hairspray, shampoo, and toothpaste have certain risk factors.

If you have allergies, exposure to toxic chemicals can aggravate those symptoms. We always blame pollen and nature's plant life for those days when we can't seem to stop sneezing and taking antihistamines. Often the culprit is right there at home with you. So many common symptoms are related to household chemicals: headaches, depression, even ordinary flu symptoms could be from an aerosol can that you used that day. Over a long period of time, toxic chemicals can contribute to cancer, birth defects, genetic changes, and many other problems. Our greatest exposure to toxic substances is not out in the industrial world in some chemical plant that most of us rarely visit. It's right in our safe little cozy homes, and every toxic chemical that we use at home eventually ends up in our environment. That chemical in the environment ultimately returns to affect us in some way. It is a vicious cycle. With everyone contributing to this, we don't know yet what the long-term effects will be.

Of the forty-eight thousand chemicals listed by the EPA, less than one thousand have been tested for immediate acute effects, and only about five hundred for their long-term effects for problems such as birth defects and genetic disorders. We know almost nothing about close to 80 percent of these chemicals and what their long-term effects could be. We have barely scratched the surface testing the synergistic effects of some of these products. The more studies that *are* actually done, the more we realize that some of the substances we once thought were safe are actually toxic to some degree. Formaldehyde resin has been found to be a factor that causes insomnia. The funny thing is that formaldehyde resin is a common ingredient in many popular wrinkle-free products used on *bedsheets*! (And you thought it was your husband's snoring.)

In many cases, toxic chemicals are manufactured from substances that are found in nature and often are labeled as "natural." That doesn't mean that they're not toxic. In fact, some of the products that are made from nature are chosen because their use in nature is toxic, such as plant and animal substances that are excreted to protect against predators. Petrochemical derivatives of crude oil are used in the majority of our industrial and consumer products. We've taken something in nature and processed it into something that is no longer natural.

The amount of synthetic organic chemicals that the United States produces in just one month is equal to the combined body weight of the 280 million people living here. In total, that's about 12 trillion pounds.

When professionals use chemicals in the workplace, they must follow very strict safety codes, thanks to government organizations like OSHA, yet we use some of the same chemicals at home and don't even know about these safety codes, much less use them.

Hearing these warnings can be overwhelming and discouraging. We do our best to eat right and exercise, only to find a whole new potentially dangerous area that needs our attention. It reminds me of comedian Jackie Mason's routine in which he says, "Scientists have now realized that everything in life kills you. Everything you do in your life is a danger to your health. No matter which direction you turn, you're in danger. So it becomes a question of picking a sickness that you like."

Take heart, guys. Jackie Mason is a one of the world's great comedians, but thank goodness he's not a doctor or a scientist. Some choices are definitely better and much safer than others are. Remember, once again, that we are a work in progress. There will *always* be obstacles to overcome. This one is not as overwhelming as it may seem at first, as long as you realize that you're not going to correct the entire problem over a weekend. Think of this as a long-term learning process of switching dangerous products with safer ones.

There are so many natural, milder, and safer alternatives that work as well and sometimes better than what you're using now. In fact, there is one product called Mother's Little Miracle that I use all the time. It's a stain and odor remover and prewash. It's completely safe around children and it's better than any other stain remover and prewash I've ever used. Also, just as there are health food stores that specialize in wholesome and natural products, there are companies providing alternative products that strive to be *chemical free*. So the task of making your house and kitchen safer doesn't have to be that difficult. Step 1 should be *awareness*. Start reading every label of your household products, just as you now read every label of your food products.

Any good science teacher will warn his class not to combine household cleaning products because you can't possibly know what new chemical combination is being created; it could be lethal. It seems strange, then, to ignore the potential chemistry lab that lurks under most of our sinks.

My mother and a friend were cleaning the floor of our dancing school and thought it would be a good idea to combine two different cleaning solutions for extra punch. I walked in to get something and noticed that both of them had watery eyes and runny noses. We immediately opened all the windows and turned on a fan, but their symptoms continued to get worse so I rushed them to the hospital. The doctor told them that they had created a highly toxic solution by combining two similar but different chemicals that could have killed them just from inhalation. They were still sick even after heavy doses of oxygen and water. Since then, I realized that common household products should never be combined and warning labels must be read carefully.

The following lists provide kitchen hazards and their safer and more natural alternatives. I urge you to read them. You may be saving your life.

KITCHEN HAZARDS

Ammonia *(also known as ammonium chloride, ammonium hydroxide, benzalkonium chloride, ammonium compounds)*

An irritant that affects the skin, eyes, and respiratory passages. It is extremely toxic when inhaled in concentrated vapors and repeated exposure may lead to bronchitis and pneumonia. It can cause chemical burns, cataracts, and corneal damage, and has been shown to produce skin cancer. Disruptions to the ecosystem can result, with toxic effects to plants, animals, and fish. The EPA lists ammonia as a toxic chemical on its Community Right-to-Know list. Found in a wide range of household cleaning products including glass cleaners, all-purpose cleaners, disinfectants, and more.

Amyl Acetate *(banana oil, pear oil)*

A skin irritant and neurotoxin causing central nervous system depression. Found in furniture polish, nail finishes, nail polish remover, and perfume.

Benzalkonium Chloride

Carcinogenic. Harmful amounts may be absorbed through skin. Irritating to mucous membranes, poisonous when ingested. Inhalation of fumes may be toxic. Cited by the EPA and OSHA as a threat to public health. Found in disinfecting hand soaps, dishwashing detergent, disinfectants, and cleaners.

Benzene

A synthetic disinfectant and bacteriacide. Wide use is causing new strains of resistant bacteria. Negatively affects living organisms. Found in oven cleaners, detergents, furniture polish, spot removers, and nail polish remover.

Butyl Cellosolve *(also known as 2-butoxy-1-ethanol, ethylene gly-*

A highly toxic synthetic solvent and grease cutter that can irritate mucous

col monobutyl ether, bu-
toxyethanol, butyl oxitol)

membranes and cause liver damage. It
is readily absorbed through the skin and
is neurotoxic. Found in some all-purpose
cleaners and degreasers, window cleaners, and a wide range of other household cleaning products.

Chlorine *(also known as sodium
hypochlorite, hypochlorite, chlorine dioxide, sodium dichloroixo-
cyanurate, hydrogen chloride, hydrochloric acid)*

A powerful irritant that can be fatal upon
inhalation. This toxic chemical causes
the most household poisonings in the
U.S., and ranks first in industrial injuries
and deaths. There is growing evidence
that chlorinated drinking water causes
bladder cancer and rectal cancer. Many
chlorinated water supplies probably contain some amount of THM (trihalo-
methanes, not Total Health Makeover!),
which are carcinogenic compounds.
THMs can be removed from tap water
with an adequate home filtration system
with activated carbon. Chlorine and compounds are environmentally damaging,
break down slowly in the ecosystem, are
stored in the fatty tissue of wildlife, and
are a prime cause of atmospheric ozone
loss. Chlorine is listed in the 1990 Clean
Air Act as a hazardous air pollutant.
Found in a wide range of household
cleaners, including laundry bleach, dishwasher detergent, tub and tile cleaners.

Cocamide DEA *(also known as
cocamide diethanolamine)*

While not carcinogenic, it has the potential to form carcinogenic nitrosamines.
Found in dishwashing liquids, sham-
poos, and cosmetics.

Colors and Dyes—*FD&C or D&C*

Artificial colors are made from petroleum and coal tar and are believed to be
cancer-causing agents. They may pene-
trate the skin, can cause allergies, and
are irritants to the skin and eyes. They
are found on labels as FD&C or D&C and

are followed by a color and number. Yellow, amber, green, or blue products are obviously dyed with synthetic colors and should be avoided.

Crystalline Silica

Eye, skin, and lung irritant, and is carcinogenic. Found in some highly popular brands of all-purpose cleaners.

D-limonene

Eye and skin irritant. Evidence of carcinogenicity. Neurotoxicity. Found in some paints, pet flea-control products, lice treatments, and some cleaning products.

DEA *(also known as di-ethanolamine, triethanolamine, and monoethanolamine)*

Moderate skin and severe eye irritant. Can react with nitrites to form carcinogenic nitrosamines. Found in a wide range of household cleaning and personal care products.

Dioxane *(also known as diethylene dioxide, diethylene ether, diethylene oxide)*

A carcinogen. It is listed as a hazardous air pollutant in the 1990 Clean Air Act. Found in window cleaners.

EDTA *(also known as ethylene-diaminetra acetic, diammonium EDTA)*

Can be an irritant to the skin and mucous membranes, leading to allergies, asthma, and skin rashes. It does not readily biodegrade and binds with heavy metals trapped in our lakes and streams, thereby activating the metals and causing them to reenter the food chain. Found in laundry detergent.

Formaldehyde

Irritating, allergy-producing, a neurotoxin and carcinogen. Can cause insomnia, coughing, headaches, nausea, nosebleeds, and skin rashes. Some of the most irritating and allergenic preservatives contain, release, or break down into formaldehyde. These include 2-bromo-2-nitropropane-1, 3-diol, diazo-

lidinyl urea, DMDM hydantoin, imidazo-
lidinyl urea, and quaternium 15. Widely
used in deodorizers, disinfectants, personal care products (including shampoo), and cosmetics (including nail polish and hardeners). A common air
pollutant, it is also used in permanent
press sheets, mattresses, foam, plas-
tics, and building materials.

Germicides

Most synthetic bacteriacides. See benzalkonium chloride. Found in disinfecting hand soaps, dishwashing detergent,
disinfectants, and cleaners.

Glycol Ether

Name for a large group of chemicals.
Can cause irritation of the skin, eyes,
nose, and throat, and some are hazardous to the reproductive system. Can
range from relatively nontoxic to extremely toxic. Can damage the kidney,
liver, and central nervous system. Can
be absorbed quickly through the skin.
Found in some household cleaning products, paints, cosmetics, and perfumes.

Hydrochloric Acid

Can dissolve and destroy tender tissues
upon direct contact. Eyes, nose, and
throat easily irritated by vapors. Can
burn, resulting in permanent scarring
and even blindness. Found in aluminum
cleaners and rust removers.

Kerosene (also mineral spirits)

Eye and skin irritant, can damage lung
tissues. Neurotoxic. May contain the carcinogen benzene. Found in all-purpose
cleaners, furniture polishes, and waxes.

Methanol (also known as methyl
alchohol)

Severe eye and skin irritant. Can cause
blindness. Neurotoxic. Found in glass
cleaners, some paint removers and
strippers, and art products.

Morpholine

Extremely toxic. Irritating to skin, eyes, and mucous membranes. May cause liver and kidney damage. Reacts with nitrites to form carcinogenic nitrosamines. Found in all-purpose cleaners, furniture polishes, and car wax.

Napthalene

Irritating to eyes and skin. Can cause cataracts, corneal damage, and kidney damage. A suspected carcinogen, extremely toxic to small children and infants. Can cause blood damage to the fetus. Found in mothballs, air fresheners, deodorizers, carpet cleaners, and toilet bowl cleaners.

Optical Brighteners

Can cause allergic reaction. Do not readily biodegrade. Toxic to fish. Found in laundry detergents.

Organic Solvents *(also known as carbon disulfide, n-hexane, metyl n-butyl ketone, trichloroethylene, perchloroethylene, toluene)*

Neurotoxic and central nervous system depressant. Many are recognized as carcinogens and reproductive hazards in the workplace. Found in all-purpose cleaners, degreasers, metal polishes, varnish and lacquer removers, dry-cleaning chemicals, paints and coatings, and adhesives.

Para-dichlorobenzene *(also known as p-dichlorobenzene, PDCB, 1,4-dichlorobenzene)*

Extremely toxic. Carcinogenic. Highly volatile. Causes liver and kidney damage. Does not biodegrade. Found in moth repellents, toilet deodorizers, room deodorants, and insecticides.

Perchloroethylene

Animal carcinogen, suspected human carcinogen. Air pollutant. Groundwater contaminant. Drinking water contaminated with perc has leukemia and birth defect implications. Long-term overexposure may affect the nervous system. Found in spot removers, degreasers, and dry-cleaning fluids.

Petroleum Distillates *(also known as naphthas)*

A group of chemicals obtained from the petroleum refining process. Eye, skin, and respiratory irritant. Neurotoxic effects can lead to organic brain damage. Many petroleum products are carcinogenic. Found in heavy-duty cleaners, laundry stain removers, furniture polish, car waxes, lice shampoo, home and garden pesticides, and pet flea-control products.

Phenol *(also known as alkyl phenoxy polyethoxy ethanol, nonyl phenoxy ethoxylate)*

Very toxic and suspected carcinogen. Swelling, pimples, and hives are common. Internal consumption can cause circulatory collapse, convulsions, cold sweats, coma, and death. Found in laundry detergent, all-purpose cleaners, air fresheners, disinfectants, and furniture polish.

Phosphates

Cause an excessive growth in aquatic plants (especially algae), leading to suffocation of fish and other aquatic life. Found in laundry detergent, dishwasher detergent, and all-purpose cleaners.

Phosphoric Acid

Eye, skin, and respiratory irritant. Breathing vapors can make lungs burn. Found in bathroom cleaners.

Propellants *(propane, butane)*

Known to cause lung diseases. Can cause eye injury and chemical burns. Found in a wide range of aerosol products, including oven cleaners, furniture polishes, air fresheners, insecticides, and personal care products.

Pyrethrin

Allergic. Neurotoxic. Found in head lice treatments, house and garden pesticides, and flea-control products.

Sodium Bisulfate

Corrosive and damaging to the eyes, skin, and internal tissues if swallowed. Can cause asthma attacks. Found in toilet bowl cleaners and deoderizers.

Sodium Hydroxide (*also known as lye, caustic soda, soda lye*)

Corrosive. Eye, skin, and respiratory irritant. Can burn eyes, skin, and internal organs. Can cause lung damage and blindness and be fatal if swallowed. Found in a wide range of household cleaners, including oven cleaners, tub and tile cleaners, toilet bowl cleaners, and drain openers.

Sodium Metasilicate

A severe eye, skin, and respiratory irritant. Inhalation can cause throat and lung damage. Found in laundry detergents and dishwasher detergents.

Stoddard Solvent

Eye and mucous membrane irritant. Neurotoxic. Found in all-purpose cleaners, abrasives, and floor and auto wax.

Sulfuric Acid

Very corrosive, producing severe burns on contact. Found in toilet bowl cleaners and metal polishes.

TEA (*also known as triethanolamine*)

Moderate skin and severe eye irritant. Can react with nitrites to form carcinogenic nitrosamines. Found in a wide range of household cleaning and personal care products.

Toluene (*also known as xylene*)

Highly toxic petrochemical solvent. Eye and skin irritant, carcinogenic, neurotoxic, and has reproductive effects. Found in spot removers, car cleaners, and paints.

Trichloroethylene (*TCE*)

Suspected carcinogen. Very irritating to eyes and nose. Found in spot removers and metal polishes.

BETTER BATHROOM BUFFERS AND CHEMICAL-FREE KITCHEN CLEANERS

Automatic Dish Detergent

Mix ½ cup baking soda with ¼ cup liquid dishwashing detergent.

Bathtub and Shower Cleaner

Using an old pair of nylons for scrubbing, make paste from cream of tartar and hydrogen peroxide. Disinfect with vinegar and old toothbrushes. Clean shower nozzles by placing them in equal parts vinegar and water, bring to boil, and let simmer 5 minutes. Clean soap scum with baby oil and damp cloth once a week. Clean caulking with bleach and water and get tight spots with rubbing alcohol and toothpick.

Chrome Polish

Use apple cider vinegar. Or try club soda in a spray bottle and crumpled aluminum foil.

Cookware Cleaner

To clean stained cookware (Pyrex and Corningware), fill a large pot or pan with water and drop in 6 Alka-Seltzer tablets. Let it soak for 1 hour, then clean. For pots and pans, fill them with white vinegar and let stand 30 minutes, then rinse in hot soapy water. Clean food graters with an old toothbrush. Make cleaning easier by spraying first with no-stick cooking spray before grating.

Copper Cleaner

Rub with lemon; rinse and dry. Or use equal parts Gold Medal flour and salt; add 1 teaspoon white vinegar to make a paste. Spread a thick layer on copper and let dry. Rinse and wipe off. Scrub and rinse with salt and lemon juice. Clean tarnish with tomato paste.

Countertop Cleaner

Scrub club soda directly onto counter, wipe with a soft cloth, rinse with warm water, and wipe dry. Buff countertops with a sheet of wax paper.

Cutting Board Cleaner

Clean and deodorize with baking soda sprinkled on a damp sponge. Rub board and rinse. To eliminate smell of garlic, onions, or fish, rub with lemon juice.

Drain Cleaner

Pour in 1 cup each baking soda and vinegar, wait 2 minutes, add 2 quarts boiling water, and repeat. Unclog drains by dropping 3 Alka-Seltzer tablets in standing water; let sit overnight.

Glass and Mirror Cleaner

Use organic potato buds mixed with enough water to make a thick paste. Cover the glass with the paste and let it sit for 24 hours, then wipe off. Try cleaning with a coffee filter.

Grill Cleaner

Make cleaning easier by rubbing with corn oil before cooking. Clean the grill after each use when it is cool to the touch.

Linoleum Cleaner

Mix 1 cup white vinegar and 2 gallons water.

Mold and Mildew Remover

Use bleach or equal parts vinegar and salt; scrub hard.

Oven Cleaner

Mix 2 tablespoons each liquid soap, borax, and warm water (cover floor of oven with aluminum foil; clean spills promptly).

Porcelain Cleaner

Pour club soda over fixtures or scrub with cream of tartar.

Tarnish Cleaner

Clean copper pots by rubbing with ketchup or tomato paste, then rinsing off. Or try rubbing Worcestershire sauce into pot with a soft cloth. Also, you can make a paste with salt and lemon juice. Scrub gently and rinse with water.

Tile Cleaner

Scrub with baking soda and damp sponge. For more abrasion, use Epsom salts mixed with castile soap or dish detergent.

Toilet Bowl Cleaner

Use baking soda and castile soap. Alka-Seltzer also works; place 2 tablets in toilet, wait 20 minutes, scrub, and flush. Any soda with citric acid will also work by leaving it in for 1 hour, then brushing and flushing. Try using 1 cup white vinegar for 5 minutes, then flush.

Water Softener

Use ¼ cup vinegar.

Wooden Salad Bowl Revitalizer

Rub with vegetable shortening inside and out and let sit overnight. Remove excess with paper towels. Wash and dry thoroughly with warm water, then rub entire bowl with a sheet of wax paper.

LIFESAVING LAUNDRY LIFTERS

Ink Spot Remover	Cold water and 1 tablespoon cream of tartar and lemon juice.
Oil Stain Remover	White chalk rubbed into stain before laundering
Perspiration Stain Remover	White vinegar and water
Scuff Mark Remover	Use a white grainy toothpaste. Apply with tissue, rub, and wipe off.
Stain Remover	Club soda, lemon juice, or salt

HEALTHY HELPERS FOR THE HOUSEHOLD

Air Freshener	Use herbal bouquets, put pure vanilla on a cotton ball, or simmer cinnamon and cloves. Purchase "light rings" for lightbulbs and put a drop of essential oil in each one. Burn orange peels.
Car Battery Corrosion Removal	Baking soda and water
Drawer Lubricator	Chapstick
Fertilizer	Compost yard clippings and organic waste from the kitchen (no meat or grease).
Pet Odor Removal	Cider vinegar
Rug and Carpet Cleaner	To deodorize, sprinkle with baking soda and let stand for 15 minutes, then vacuum. Get spots out with ¼ cup Murphy's oil soap. Get coffee out with Huggies baby wipes.
Rusty Bolt and Nut Remover	Carbonated beverages

Window Cleaner

Use 2 tablespoons vinegar in 1 quart water. Or fill a spray bottle with club soda and use a pair of nylons (also works on window screens).

Wood Cleaner

To fix scratches, rub with soy or Worcestershire sauce until achieving the right tone of brown. To get rid of white rings on furniture, apply Nayonaise. Let stand an hour, wipe off, and polish. To clean varnished wood, hand-buff with a towel shoved into one leg of nylons. Cold Lipton tea is a good cleaning agent for any kind of woodwork.

CONTROLLING CREEPY CRITTERS

Ants

Sprinkle crushed red pepper or chili powder where you find the ants entering. Try drawing a line of Crayola chalk around windows and doors of your home and around water pipes inside your home. They won't cross a chalk line. Gold Medal flour also works if you fill cracks and make a line where ants enter. They won't cross through. Or put vinegar in a spray bottle or mister with an equal part water and spray around doorjambs, windowsills, water pipes, and foundation cracks. Dried coffee will work if placed outside doors and cracks. Coffee deters ants.

Bees, Wasps, and Yellow Jackets

Fill an empty jar with one can of beer. Punch ⅜-inch holes in the lid and cover tightly. Place near plants where insects pollinate. They love it and drown in it. What a way to go. Syrup-coated cardboard around the perimeter of the yard will keep them away.

Fleas	Gradually add brewer's yeast to your pet's diet (consult your veterinarian). Or apply a little eucalyptus oil on the neck of the animal. Wash the doghouse with salt water to keep them away.
Flies	Put out a well-watered bowl of basil. Invest in a fly swatter. Hang a Kleenex tissue on a string on a screen door to scare them away.
Mealworms	Place a few sticks of wrapped Wrigley's spearmint gum on a shelf near open packages of pasta. Spearmint repels them.
Mosquitoes	Burn citronella candles or oil.
Moths	Place a few cedar chips in cotton sachets and place in closet or drawers. Or put black pepper in a cheesecloth bag or foot of nylon as a sachet.
Plant Insects	Rub soapy water on leaves, then rinse.
Repellent	A little vinegar on the skin will repel the bugs.
Roaches	Leave chopped bay leaves and cucumber skins in strategic places.
Slugs and Snails	Kill with one can of beer in an open jar. They drown in it.

3

In with the
Good Stuff!

I have always considered Wednesday, August 15, 1979, my health birthday, because it was on that day that I made the firm commitment to give up the Big Three: meat, sugar, and dairy. Earlier in the day, I had gone to a nutritionist for the first time. He was a full medical doctor who specialized in natural medicine, herbs, and supplements. Based on my family history and a full examination (including "reading my face"), he suggested that I give up meat, sugar, and dairy products.

My first step as a non-meat/non-sugar/ non-dairy person was to go shopping at a major health food store for the first time. I remember hearing that there was this great store in Los Angeles called Erewhon. At first, I was a little intimidated to go to this strange new place, but when I pulled up in front, I saw a tall, dark, and handsome Erewhon regular whom I knew well, Jeff Goldblum. Jeff and I had worked together in a film a few years before, and I had always found him to be fun, healthy, and full of energy. He told me that he shopped at Erewhon all the time and would be happy to show me around. I explained to him that this was my first time, but he reassured me that he would be "gentle."

Jeff was so wonderful that day! He took me through each and every aisle and pointed out the healthiest and best-tasting products to buy. He told me about the ones I shouldn't buy as well. He even taught me about buying in bulk. It was the perfect introduction to the world of health food. I've run into Jeff several times since then, and I always tell him how grateful I am that he had de-(white)-floured me that day and how he's such a terrific guy. Because I had this wonderful knight in shining armor to guide me through my first experience in a health food store, I decided that I would do likewise for all of my friends who wanted the same. And that's what I'm going to do for you in this chapter.

A Walk Through a Health Food Store

Our journey begins at Whole Foods Market in Los Angeles. One of the reasons I wanted to give this tour at Whole Foods is because Whole Food Markets are all over the country. Even if you're an old pro at this, join me on this venture anyway. I promise you'll discover something new.

Aisle Foods

The first thing I'm seeing as I walk in is **coffee**. Now, I'm not a coffee drinker. I gave it up years ago. But if you're going to drink coffee, try to drink decaffeinated, and make it water-pressed decaf rather than a coffee where the caffeine is chemically bleached out. You might also want to look at some of the coffee alternatives. Roma is wonderful. It's a natural grain beverage that satisfies that gotta-have-something-warm-in-the-morning feeling. It's more like a coffee than a tea.

At the bakery section, I see a lot of great **breads**. As you probably already know, I don't believe you need to give up bread on this program. The main thing to do when choosing a bread is to avoid one that is overprocessed and/or contains refined sugar and dairy products. There are so many types of breads that you can choose from, especially if you can get them fresh at the bakery section of your supermarket or health food store. No matter which bread you buy, packaged or fresh, carefully read the label of each one, because even a conscientious store like Whole Foods carries breads with some preservatives, refined sugar, and dairy products. Don't ever assume that a product automatically doesn't have preservatives, refined sugar, or dairy products in it just because it's sold at a health food store.

My favorite brand of bread sold at most health food stores is by Food for Life. Their raisin bread and Ezekiel 4:9 Whole Grain Bread are especially good. I used to love Squaw Bread, but it now contains dairy products—so make sure that you read the labels to be certain the ingredients haven't changed. There are many terrific breads and whole-grain products in this section, such as **muffins**, **bagels**, multigrain and whole rye and olive breads. Even when I was traveling throughout Europe, and having a hard time finding a health food store, I could always find whole-grain rye breads in regular local supermarkets. I love the really strong-flavored little **flatbreads** that look like brownstone bricks. I found them all over Europe, and luckily they're now common here, too. These breads are delicious and have a rich hearty texture. Slice by slice, you really can taste the rye flavor. (It's amazing how delicious something this simple can taste after you've really cleaned up your palate!) If you compare the ingredients of a loaf of white bread to a loaf of whole-grain bread, you'd be shocked. They don't even seem like the same type of product. Everything that is vibrant and healthy has been completely bleached out of the white bread.

One of the best ways to find a product that is safe to eat is to look for one that is labeled **vegan**. In order for a product to earn a vegan label it has to be made without animal products. It usually means a minimal amount of processing as well. Twenty-one years ago, when I started eating this way, I could barely find anything healthy to eat in a regular grocery store. And what I did find in a health food store was often hippy-dippy-looking and not always fresh. But now there are so many great products.

I'm standing in front of the **cookie** section, and dying right now because I see Uncle Eddie's Vegan Cookies. If you want a great pleasure-food cookie with no sugar and no dairy, but that's still sinfully delicious, this is your cookie. Although they are not fat-free, they are lower in calories and fat content than other wicked cookies that you'll find in conventional stores. Uncle Eddie's Vegan Cookies are outrageously good. They come in four different flavors and couldn't be better.

They fool all of my junk-food-eating friends. I always bring them to kids' birthday parties or to school whenever I'm asked to bring a treat. No one ever believes that there is no refined sugar or dairy in these cookies. (Oh my gosh, I'm beginning to sound like I'm on commission!)

Speaking of sinful, I'm now looking at **chocolate**. People say to me, "Isn't chocolate always made with milk or yogurt or whey?" I tell them that you can buy chocolate that has no dairy whatsoever. It does have cocoa butter, but that's not dairy butter. Some of the chocolate products found at Whole Foods have refined sugar, and some don't. Once again, make sure you read the label. One of the best brands is Tropical Source.

Okay, the next section I'm walking through is the **cheese** section and I have to hold my nose because it smells like body parts to me (one particular body part, in fact—feet!). It smells horrible. I can't believe I used to like that smell.

Next is the **deli** section. Whenever you're in a deli or in the deli section of your grocery store, you should not be afraid to ask the deli person to tell you the ingredients in any item. Don't be intimidated. He will know what he prepared and will probably have a list of all the ingredients. If he doesn't know for sure, ask to see the master recipe book that every restaurant or deli keeps in order to ensure uniformity in the recipes. You may be surprised at how helpful and informative deli servers can be. Freshness is important, too. You should also ask how recently something was prepared. Asking for this kind of information is not at all out of line. You should know what you're putting in your body every single day.

In the **soy cheese** section, you've got to be really careful. Some soy cheeses are great, and some are horrible. Soya Kaas is one of the better ones. It tastes good and is great for cooking because it melts well, but know that their fat-free brand doesn't work at all. I would stick to the regular Soya Kaas or their veggie singles. I would also recommend Soyco's Lite & Less Veggie Slices for its taste and "meltability" (the favorite for grilled "cheese" sandwiches!). And it comes in a variety of flavors, including Swiss, provolone, and pepper jack. The different flavors of Lisanatti's Soy Sensation and RiceSlice are good and they melt well, too. Of the various grated Parmesan-style soy cheeses, my favorite is Lite and Less. Soya Kaas and Rice Parmesan I would recommend second. But forget the fat-free versions of any of these brands.

Tofu comes in two different styles: silken (good for baking) and in water (great for marinating and frying). And each style comes in three different forms: soft, firm, and extra firm. Of the different brands of tofu, Nasoya, White Wave, and Nori are all excellent. Each brand comes in all six versions.

My favorite company that uses soy to make **meat substitute** products is Yves. They don't use sugar, dairy, or meat in any of their products, including **tofu wieners, veggie wieners, chili dogs, jumbo veggie dogs, ground round, pepperoni slices, soy turkey,** and **burgers** of all kinds. You name it, they do it. They have taken this art form to a new level. My favorite of all is their **veggie breakfast links**. I always loved **sausages** as a child. It was one of the hardest things for me to give up, but because of this product, I can always get my sausage fix. Litelife's Gimme Lean and Hamburger **Chili** are also great.

Here in California, we eat a lot of **guacamole**. If you don't have time to make your own from avocados, or if you live in a place where avocados are out of season, try Señor Felix's Guacamole. You can determine the degree of spiciness because they put the salsa on top; you can mix in all of it, some of it, or none of it. Another great product is Vegenaise, from Follow Your Heart. It's a **mayonnaise** substitute. Although it has the same fat content as mayonnaise, it has none of the bad stuff, has a great texture, and is one of the best mayonnaise substitutes I've ever tasted. It's worth mentioning here, however, that Nayonaise, which is not in the refrigerated section of your health food store, is the mayonnaise substitute we use most often because it is a soy product and has one-third the amount of fat of regular mayonnaise.

One product that I highly recommend you buy is **miso**. It is a salty soybean paste that can be used to make spreads, sauces, and soups. There are many excellent brands such as Miso Master, Westbrae, and Cold Mountain. Miso is a staple of healthy cooking. It has saved me many times. Miso soup is great for settling my kids' stomachs (or anyone's) whenever they're not feeling well. You can make it instantly by adding a teaspoon of miso paste to 2 cups of hot water, not boiled. Never boil miso. Boiling kills most of the good enzymes.

In the **boxed beverage** section, look for Rice Dream. We use Rice Dream for everything—drinking, cooking, and baking. Original Enriched is the flavor most like milk. In fact, we even make mashed potatoes with it. I'm a big, big fan of Imagine Foods, which is the manufacturer. My kids were raised on Rice Dream **drinks, puddings,** and **frozen bars**. Imagine has just come out with a new drink called Power Dream, which is a **power drink**. Their boxed Soy Dream and West Soy's Plus are both great for baking, especially when you want a creamy texture.

Other great boxed **soy milks** are by EdenSoy (Eden also sells a rice and soy blend), and Soy Moo (sold at Trader Joe's).

Next, the **boxed juice drink** section. Unfortunately, many parents will go out and pick any brand of juice, but many of these products have high-fructose corn syrup, refined sugar, Nutrasweet, or something else added that's just as bad. Make sure you read the label. It's very important that you get 100 percent **juice**. One of the greatest boxed juices that my boys and I have fallen in love with is called Vroot. It comes in a variety of blends, including tropical, orange veggie, and berry veggie. Vroot also comes in small sizes so you can pack them in your kids lunchboxes. Knudsen and Ceres also contain 100 percent juice. Remember, you've got to read the label carefully even when you're buying at a health food store. Another great juice I would recommend for children is from After The Fall. They have different flavors and you can find this brand all over the country. I discovered After The Fall when I was living in New York twenty years ago, so I know this company has been around for a long time. It's reputable and its flavors are great.

Okay, now I'm in the **spice rack.** Whole Foods has its own line of spices, and there are other great products as well. Spice Hunter, Frontier, Spike, Vegisol, and Onion Magic are all good products. Spike is a great **salt substitute**. To find the spices and flavor enhancers that will work for you, it is best to read the labels carefully and do a lot of your own experimenting. It can be a real adventure. You'll end up with a few clinkers along the way, but I'm sure you'll find some gems as well. A wonderful spice that you can buy or make yourself is **gomasio**. Mix fifteen parts sesame seeds to one part salt. This makes a great flavor enhancer. I learned about it when I first began studying macrobiotics in the seventies. My kids love it, and it's a great source of calcium. It's a wonderful way to get a lot of flavor while using a very limited amount of salt.

As far as sweet food enhancers are concerned, the best brand is Tropical Source **chocolate chips**. We use a lot of these in our dessert recipes for things like chocolate chip cookies and muffins. They now have peanut-butter-chocolate chips and espresso-chocolate-flavored chips along with their regular chocolate-flavored chips. All of them are without sugar and dairy. They taste better than the chips you are used to using. (You can imagine how much my kids love them!)

Speaking of kids, there are plenty of **dessert puddings** available. Imagine Foods' chocolate, banana, butterscotch, and lemon puddings are outstanding! I guarantee your kids will eat them. I put them in my kids' lunch boxes, and I serve them often when it's my turn to bring in the snack at their school. The other kids never guess that there's no sugar or dairy in them. Imagine Foods has done it again. Another company that's very good is Lundberg. They also have dairy-free and sugar-free puddings.

One of the best companies for **flour** is Arrowhead Mills. They have many different flours and have kept all the good stuff in them: **oat flour, whole wheat flour, rye flour**. Even their white pastry flour is whole grain. Arrowhead Mills also makes **biscuit** and **pancake mixes.** These are also non-sugar, non-dairy. Always read the labels to make sure. Products change.

For **cooking oils**, I recommend Spectrum. They offer a pretty big variety of oils: sesame, corn, safflower, as well as other oils. Also, there are plenty of sprays that you'll find in a health food store. There's even a spray called Butter Delight that has a butter flavor that is all natural, is made out of vegetable oil, and contains no dairy. It's made by Tryson House. They also offer Olive Mist, Oriental Mist, and Italian Mist.

For **applesauces** and other **fruit products** that come in jars, like **jams** and **jellies**, read the label to make sure no sugar is added. Fruit is already so sweet. I have never understood why sugar and/or corn syrup are often added to these products. Trust me, your kids will love them more than the jellies with sugar, especially after their palates adjust. A lot of these products are organic, so don't settle for products that are not. Whole Foods sells their own line. Other good brands are Sorrell Ridge, Santa Cruz, Newton family, and Leroux Creek. These are great for your child's lunch box.

Next, I'd like to talk about packaged **grains** like **tabouli, hummus, falafel,** and **rice**. One of my favorite brands is Kasbah, and my kids love all of their pilafs: **nutted pilaf, rice pilaf,** and their **lentil pilaf**. Near East and Fantastic are other good companies. Barbara's carries a lot of good products like their **mashed potatoes,** but you have to read Barbara's labels carefully, because some of them list sugar and dairy.

Oatmeal is one of my favorite things to eat and serve for breakfast. We usually get Erewhon oatmeal because it is so quick and easy and comes in so many different flavors, but Arrowhead Mills, Lundberg, Mother's, and (especially) McCann's Irish Oatmeal are also fantastic.

We use a lot of **sugar substitutes** in the recipes in this book. (For more information and a complete chart, see Chapter 4, page 72). **Sucanat** and **Rapadura** are made from evaporated whole cane juice. With this type of process, the minerals and molasses are retained. Evaporation differs from the process used to make refined white sugar, which removes 98 percent of the nutrients. Sucanat and Rapadura are great sweeteners. Sucanat is easy to use and has a really rich flavor. Use it whenever you would normally use sugar. Turbinado and raw sugar often claim to be in the same category, but they are not. **Date sugar** is made from ground and dehydrated dates. Use it as you would white sugar. Try using it in combination with other sweeteners. Date sugar has a somewhat hearty flavor. **Honey,** as everyone knows, is extracted from flower nectar by bees. Colors and tastes vary depending on the flower source. It is sweeter than white sugar, so use less. **Maple sugar** (my favorite) is dehydrated maple syrup and has a nice rich flavor. Use it in all baked goods as you would white or brown sugar. There is also **barley malt syrup**, which is made from sprouted barley. It is dark brown and dense. It tastes a little bit like molasses but is not as sweet as white sugar, so you have to use more to get the same effect. **Brown rice syrup** is made from brown rice and various enzymes. It has an amber color and mild butterscotch flavor. Use it in recipes for cookies, pies, and puddings.

Sugar substitutes all have different flavors and textures and it can be fun trying to find out what sweetener works best in your favorite recipes. There is definitely no reason to ever use refined white sugar again. My favorite brand names are Lundberg brown rice syrup, Whole Foods or Shady Maple Farms **maple syrup**, Knudsen or plantation concentrates, Barbados unsulfured **molasses**, and Bernard Jensen's **rice bran syrup**. His products are always very good and really healthy.

Now let's move on to **peanut butters** and other **nut butters**. One Christmas, my husband and I gave everybody a large assortment of nut butters and **jellies**. The nut butters were from Marantha Nut Butters. They come in macadamia, cashew, almond, et cetera. You name it! And they are delicious! The jellies were from Sorrell Ridge, which makes its jellies from 100 percent fruit. Remember—you don't need jelly that has anything in it but 100 percent fruit, so read the label.

For **cold cereals**, my kids like a lot of different brands, but I'd have to say that the three most popular cereals in my family are Puffins, Shredded Spoonfuls, and Fruity Punch. Actually, my boys like these three so much they made up their own recipe called "Slip Slop Cereal," which is all three mixed together. They also like Barbara's New Morning Os and Wafflers, which are made by U. S. Mills. Kids' favorites change monthly, so I encourage you to try many different types of cereal.

Always in your health food store, there's a section that has **macrobiotic products**. It has various things you might use, like pickled ginger or daikon radish. It also has the different **seaweeds** and **sea vegetables** like kombu, nori, arame, dulse flakes, hijiki, and wakame. Each seaweed has a different texture and a slightly different flavor. You can use them in soup stocks, in salads, and to make sushi rolls. Sea vegetables are one of the healthiest things you can eat. And **umeboshi plums**. Everyone should have umeboshi plums in their refrigerator. It's part of the Healthy Life Kitchen. They are the best thing whenever you feel out of balance. They're extremely salty and they come with shiso leaves, but they are the most incredible thing if you ever have a digestion problem. You take a very little bit of it and put it on your tongue, or under your tongue. And as I told you in my first book, if you ever have motion sickness, you should tape one to your belly button. (Okay, I've now lost my entire audience.)

The **crackers** I buy most often are from Hain, Whole Foods, and Barbara's. Again, read labels carefully. Even companies that are known for making healthy products often produce a few that are questionable. Don't trust a name and buy whatever they make.

Hain and Health Valley make very good **canned products**. Bearitos and Shelton Farms do as well. Both, however, tend to use chicken and turkey in their soups and chilies. So if you don't eat poultry, be careful. Read the labels on canned goods to make sure the canning process is safe and lead-free. Twenty-one years ago, when I started this, lead-free was nearly nonexistent.

You have to really watch it with **cup-of-soup** products. Many are laden with chemicals. I have found Health Valley, Fantastic, Ramen, and Nile to have labels I can trust. These instant soups have saved me on so many film locations. They're easy to pack in a bag, and you can always get hot water. There are many different flavors, so there's no excuse for not having a healthy lunch at work. Just use the hot water reserved for tea. A company called Organic Gourmet makes a fantastic wild mushroom soup (they also make a great vegetable soup). It is an instant soup and stock. I use it in a lot of my recipes with fish or vegetables, and it's incredible. Imagine Foods makes a great line of creamy soups that have absolutely no dairy in them, like broccoli, butternut squash, mushroom, and gazpacho. Vegetable broth is used instead of chicken. Pacific Organic is a good brand name that makes boxed soups. You can store these in your cupboard until you open them. You can also take these "to go" since they don't require refrigeration.

People often say to me, "I can't be healthy at work because there's nothing but junk food in the cafeteria." Well, there's no excuse anymore! There are too many products out there that you can bring with you to work. If you truly want to feel better and be more productive every day, you have to eat a good breakfast *and* a good lunch. The last thing I want to mention is a product my kids love called **Natural Kids Meals** from Grandma Malina's Kitchen. They make organic pasta rings and veggie franks and organic veggie franks and beans.

Uh-oh. I'm facing those damn Uncle Eddie's Vegan **Cookies** again. They're located in two different sections in this store, so they really get you coming and going. (Either that, or I've just been circling hoping to run into them again.) I keep buying them, and, luckily, my brother, Lorin, keeps eating them. If you want a lighter cookie, Hain makes Honey Animal Grahams and Heaven Scent makes the old windmill cookies. Both are great! You can also get animal cookies like the ones from our childhood, except now you can give them to your children and know that they're not going to be getting refined sugar and preservatives. Always check the label, though. Another brand that my kids love is New Morning Organic Honey Grahams. They're really good. I often bring them to school for a healthy snack.

The **snack** section is one in which you have to really read the labels carefully. You have to watch especially for chemicals, fat, and sodium here. Snack companies are very tricky at disguising their fat content. Once you find a reputable company, go with it. The Good Health Company makes great **veggie sticks** that contain 40 percent less fat than potato chips. They come in three different flavors—corn, spinach, and carrot. My kids love them! They also love Fruity Booty, Veggie Booty, Ginkgo Biloba Rings, and Power Puffs with Ginseng, made by Robert's American Gourmet. Power Puffs look like the old standard **cheese puffs**, but they're non-dairy with natural ingredients and they taste better. For **popcorn**, try Bearitos. I also recommend trying Paul Newman. (His popcorn! Don't get excited! It's called Newman's Own.) Watch out with popcorn. Butter or hydrogenated oils are often used and the fat and salt content in popcorn is usually very high. **Rice cakes** are a healthy alternative to chips and buttered popcorn. Hain and Lundberg offer a wide variety of rice cakes. (My favorite is Hain's Honey Nut.) Lundberg's Rice Cakes are a little more dense, but they are really good. Fun pleasure foods don't have to be boring or unhealthy. Even **potato chips** from a health food store taste better. The typical potato chips that we grew up with are too salty and unnatural tasting once you get used to eating a product like Kettle Chips. The best products for potato chips and other snacks are Kettle Chips, Guiltless Gourmet, and Newman's Own. All three offer a wide variety.

Frozen foods have advanced the most in the health food industry during the last twenty years. The varieties today are immeasurable compared to what was offered in the seventies. Amy's is an excellent product line. They do a lot of great non-dairy dishes like tofu vegetable lasagna. Cascadian Farms is also a reputable label for frozen foods. I often buy Health Is Wealth veggie munchies and pizza supreme munchies for my boys. It's nice to buy snack foods for my kids and not have to worry about how bad it is for them or that they're going to have an energy crash in the middle of their school day.

The number one staple in our house is **soybeans**. There is always a bowl ready to eat sitting on our kitchen table for my family and guests. When friends come to visit, they will automatically (without asking) walk up and start snacking on the soybean bowl. They're not being bold or rude. They just know that's why it's there. Natural Touch makes a great soybean product. I see soybeans everywhere these days. They have recently become so popular, they were even featured in a cover story in *USA Today* not long ago. I have been bragging about soybeans for the last twenty years. The one thing to watch out for when you're buying them is to make sure you don't buy those that are genetically engineered. Because soybeans are so popular now, some companies are genetically engineering them to rush them to market. If you don't see anything on the label to help you, check with your grocer. If the label says "organic" or "not genetically engineered," it should be okay. Soybeans are not the only **frozen organic vegetable** you can buy. Cascadian Farm is a wonderful label. They have practically everything: organic garden peas, chopped spinach, sweet corn, Thai stir-fry, and even frozen French fries. When I prepare fries for my kids, I bake them in the toaster oven. I don't need to use any oil. Spud puppies are also great to prepare in the toaster oven.

Another very popular product in our home is **Boca Burgers**. We eat their veggie burgers, meatless tenders, et cetera. Lately, however, they've been slipping dairy in some of their products. This is what I mean about periodically rechecking the products you use regularly, because they will change without alerting you. Natural Touch makes some great frozen meat substitute products as well. Okara Patty is very good; people always think it's made with okra (that slimy vegetable), but it's not. And they have different flavors of black bean burgers that are very good.

Van's **Toaster Waffles** are great. They're easy to prepare, all natural, and there are several kinds: Belgian waffles, mini-waffles, organic waffles, wheat free, blueberry, and cinnamon. Some have dairy, so be careful. I love the convenience of these waffles. Healthy eating doesn't have to be a burden anymore.

Here is my kids' favorite, the **ice cream** section. My children, six and four and a half years old, have never tasted real ice cream. The truth is they're not even interested in milk-made ice cream because they enjoy the natural non-dairy ice creams so much. Rice Dream and Sweet Nothings are good, but Organic Soy Delicious is by far the best. Try vanilla and chocolate peanut butter. Be careful, though—some non-dairy ice creams can be high in fat, just like regular ice cream. Remember that we're talking about pleasure food here. But the nice thing about these pleasure foods is that you don't have to feel sick the next day. Along with rice and soy ice cream, try some of the great fruit smoothies made by Cascadian. These are healthy to eat for breakfast.

If you like **salsa chips**, try Garden of Eatin's Blue Chips, Sesame Blues, or Black Bean Chips (my boys' favorite). Whole Foods, Enrico's, and Guiltless Gourmet also make some good chips and salsas. They are all surprisingly low in fat.

My new favorite **soy yogurt,** which just last week won my Discovery-of-the-Week-Guaranteed-to-Be-Eaten-in-My-Kid's-Lunch-Box Award is Whole Soy Yogurt. It's become so popular that my local Whole Foods can barely keep it in stock. There are two other good ones, as well: Nancy's and Silk, which is made by White Wave.

If you're going to eat **eggs,** they should be free range, cage free, verified organic ONLY! Don't buy commercial eggs ever! I believe that much of the breast and ovarian cancers we're getting are from eating eggs laid by hormone- and antibiotic-injected hens. (It makes sense, doesn't it?)

When buying **olive oil**, make sure you buy cold-pressed extra-virgin olive oil imported from Italy. There are so many wonderful brands; just read the label to make sure it says "cold pressed" and "extra virgin." There are some great balsamic **vinegars,** too. Spectrum makes a great organic apple cider vinegar, and Eden makes a terrific brown rice vinegar.

For **margarine**, I recommend buying only non-hydrogenated. Hydrogenated oils have been linked in some studies to breast and colon cancer and heart disease. Neither Spectrum Spread nor Earth Balance use hydrogenated oils. And there's a new product called Rice Butter that's also non-hydrogenated. It's made from organic brown rice and it actually tastes a lot like butter.

When buying **pasta**, carefully read the label. Some of the top name-brand pastas are enriched, like DiCecco. I don't recommend you eat it every day, but it is a quality brand. There are some great organic whole-wheat pastas that are more natural and less processed. (I'll admit, they do take a little getting used to. You might have to ease into them.)

For **pasta sauce**, look for Enrico's, Newman's Own, Malina's Finest, Whole Foods brand, and Muir Glen. All are good, but I think our favorites are Enrico's and Malina's. Carefully check the labels on all brands. Some brands contain sugar and some don't.

The cooking team has really fallen in love with a few products while working on this project. One of them is Silk **soy milk**. We've been bragging about how easy it has been to use in place of milk. It comes in plain, vanilla, and chocolate.

For **salad dressings**, try Annie's, Newman's Own, Cardini's, Nasoya, Spectrum, or Whole Foods brand. They're all good. Annie's Natural is probably my favorite. It has a very fresh, real food taste. You can actually taste the flavors. If you compare the ingredients in Annie's to a popular commercial brand sold in conventional supermarkets, you'll see a big difference. The commercial brand will usually claim to be low-fat, or even no fat, but it will be completely loaded with chemicals! Of course it contains no fat! IT CONTAINS NO FOOD EITHER!

I have mentioned **Bragg Liquid Aminos** in my other books. I have received so many letters asking me, "What the heck is Bragg's?" It is natural liquid aminos (a liquid vegetable protein seasoning) made by health food pioneers Paul and Patricia Bragg. The best way for me to describe it is to read a description straight from the bottle: "Essential and non-essential amino acids in naturally occurring amounts from liquid-protein from soybeans only." It's a soy product, but it's not as strong or as salty as soy sauce. Many people use it as a salt substitute. (I even spray it on air-popped popcorn.) I think it tastes better than salt. Please try it! It may become the most important condiment in your kitchen.

For **soy sauce**, try Premiere Japan, Eden, Westbrae Natural, or Sanjay. All are very good. They have different flavorings and are great for marinating fish or chicken.

Nayonaise, used in many of the recipes in this book, has one-third the fat of mayonnaise. It's a soy product and tastes like mayonnaise, but it's so much better for you. My kids love it! In fact, they recently tasted real mayonnaise and thought the flavor was strange, probably because they've only eaten Nayonaise. Your children should be able to adjust to most of these healthier products easily, especially if they are young. Do it slowly (but surely) if you're afraid they're going to rebel. But I'm telling you, there are so many healthy products that have as much flavor as the unhealthy ones, and you'll quickly notice how less frequently your children get sick.

For **mustards**, try Westbrae Natural or Whole Foods brand. Both make quality mustards: yellow, stone ground, or Dijon.

My kids like both Westbrae Natural and Muir Glen organic tomato **ketchup**.

They taste just like the real thing. In fact, they taste better than the real thing, because what we consider to be the real thing is not the real thing! This is the real thing because this has real tomatoes in it . . . and the other . . . well . . . oh . . . You know what I mean!

When it comes to any kind of **turkey sausage** or **chicken dogs** or any other **poultry product**, the best is Shelton Farms. They're all naturally organic. They have great-tasting (so my husband claims) turkey breakfast sausage and turkey Italian sausage. He cooks with them all the time and loves just about everything Shelton Farms makes.

Now I'm in the **produce section**, the wonderful produce section. When people tell me that they have a tough time walking away from the dinner table once they get started, I tell them that for an experiment they should try for three days to eat as much as they want and as frequently as they want. The only restriction is that they must buy all of their food in the produce section. Every vitamin and nutrient is right there. In fact, most people would get more nutrients than they're getting now if they followed this restriction. I'm sure that anyone who did this once in a while would be their healthiest and look their best. This goes back to my theory that if you concentrate on the quality of what you eat, you eventually don't have to worry about the quantity. The quantity will take care of itself.

If you're at all uncertain about the different options in the produce section, the best way to learn is to ask the man who knows best, the produce man. Even if you think you know everything there is to know about fruits and vegetables, this is still a good excuse to talk to a nice handsome guy. The following is based on my interview with my two favorite produce guys.

Fruits

Apples: Apples (like people) are more appealing when they're firm. Some people hit them to see if they reverberate inside. But I'm not sure if that really works. (If you ever see someone doing this, please don't intervene. Just call the Apple Abuse Hotline.) I think it's best to simply look for apples that are solid with no bruises, cuts, or indentations. Those are all signs that they were dropped (or reverberated) and will probably turn brown inside.

Bananas: Look for the ones that are solid and golden with no discoloration or brown marks. Remember that organic bananas don't ripen after they're picked, but conventional bananas *do* ripen afterward because of the pesticide gas. There's a lot of controversy about which you should eat. I always feel that if pesticides are designed to kill bugs, they are going to be affecting your central nervous system as well.

Berries: Look for uniform color and make sure there is no mold. If you see anything that looks white on the inside, especially with raspberries, don't get them, because they're going to get moldy very soon. Avoid wet berries, too.

If you get home and realize you bought something spoiled, take it back. Nearly every store will be happy to take it back for a refund without any questions.

Coconuts: Shake them and make sure you can hear the milk inside. They shouldn't be cracked or have any mold around the eyes. That's a sign of age.

Grapes: Make sure they're firm, have a good color, and taste good. Don't be afraid to taste one or two to judge. It's perfectly fine to do this. Just don't pull up a chair and start your own picnic. You have to taste them because they can often look good yet be sour.

Oranges: Try to pick oranges that have a uniform color and aren't too soft. Softness is the first sign of decay. After that, they start to get moldy.

Pears: Watch for cuts and bruises as you do with apples.

Pineapples: Pick one that is golden, smells sweet, and has quills that can be plucked easily from the top. Most tropical fruits don't ripen up well after they're picked, so don't select one that's greener even if you're not planning to eat it for a few days. The color won't break properly, and it won't sweeten up. That is why you should also judge by smell. You can smell the ripe ones.

Organic fruits and vegetables are rarely as photogenic or as large as conventional fruit, but they're usually tastier and sweeter. Even though I'm telling you to select evenly colored, unblemished fruit, you should still choose organic. Never pick a conventional apple over an organic apple just because the conventional one is a little prettier. (Remember, beauty's only skin deep.) Sometimes, however, you'll get the best of both worlds and see beautiful *organic* vegetables and fruits. If you do, buy them immediately and throw a party! Also keep in mind, you should buy things in season. Produce breaks down faster when it's out of season. You'll find that organic produce is not even available unless it's in season. When the weather gets hot, the sugar content in all the fruits and vegetables goes up. That's why fruits and vegetables taste so much better in the summer. Buying melons in the winter is not recommended no matter where you live. Melons can be imported from the tropics, but they will not keep well once they get here. Also, when fruits and vegetables are shipped from a warm climate to a cold one, there is a transition period. Therefore, they have to be picked before they're ripe so they never have the chance to completely tree ripen. This explains the loss of flavor.

Vegetables

Broccoli: This is my favorite vegetable. Look at the crown and make sure that it's solid. You'll be able to feel it. If it's soft, it will wilt. You'll be able to see it. It will be like a sponge. Also look for one that's uniform in color. If they start turning orange or gold at all, that means they're starting to sprout and flower. You don't want them flowering. It's nice to pick one that's really dark, too. They can even be black. Simply put: think firm, solid, and a uniform dark color. My boys love the broccoli stem. I peel (like a carrot) the lower part of the stalk (that I would normally throw away), and they eat it as a healthy snack. You can even make broccoli slaw out of just the stalk or use it as an ingredient in making coleslaw.

Cabbage: A good cabbage should be fairly heavy, not too light, so you know it's dense and clean. Sometimes you have to take off the outer leaves because they may be dried up, but underneath they should be heavy and dense. They vary in color (green or red), but pick one whose color is vibrant—a nice pale green or a deep purply red.

Carrots: Root vegetables in general should be firm, solid, and have a nice color. Try bending them. If they bend too easily, it's not as desirable as when they break easily.

Cauliflower: Don't pick one that has any discoloration. Once it starts getting discolored, it's usually pretty old. Cauliflower should be white and hard.

Celery: Celery should be firm and crisp and free of bruises and blemishes.

Corn: It's best to go with the smaller kernels when selecting corn. Look at the outer leaves and make sure they're a fresh-looking green color, not yellow. You're allowed to pull the husk back if you want.

Mushrooms: Look underneath the cap to make sure they don't have any discoloration. White mushrooms should be closed before you purchase them, unlike shiitake and portobello mushrooms, which are open.

The white ones should look nice, white, and clean with no gray marks. Portobellos and shiitakes are a different story. Just make sure they're fresh and they're not dried up around the edges.

Onions: Onions should still have their skin. Their skin falling off is a sign of aging. Check the tops and the bottoms where the shoots would be. Sometimes they get soft, which means the onions are going bad.

Peppers: Pick peppers with bright and consistent color. Look for one that has a good shape for its type (anything not irregular). Avoid bruised or broken peppers.

Potatoes: Potatoes should be firm. They should not be green at all, and they should never be sprouting in any spots. There's a chemical in those sprouts that is carcinogenic. The indentations on a potato are where they will sprout. So, if they have fewer indentations, they will have less of a chance of spoiling. Those indentations are called the eyes. The fewer eyes, the better. Some people simply cut off the sprouts, but it's really not advisable to eat potatoes once they've started sprouting.

Salad Bags: If your store has a fast turnover, don't be afraid to use the pre-washed, precut salad bags. If they're fresh, go right ahead. They'll save you a lot of time. It's a good idea to wash these anyway, even though they're prewashed.

Spinach: Make sure the leaves are crisp and free of moisture. Avoid broken or browning and bruised leaves.

Sprouts: These are some of the fastest-spoiling vegetables, so buy them only a day or two before you plan to use them.

Tomatoes: Make sure that they shine. Often tomatoes are coated with an oily composite to keep them from dehydrating, but a good tomato will usually shine. It will gleam a bit. When tomatoes get older, they get dull.

Zucchinis: These should be firm and fairly shiny. Don't pick one with scratches, bump marks, or cracks.

Fish and Seafood

The most important factor when buying fish is freshness, so ask the manager of the seafood department what the "catch of the day" is. If you're planning ahead, you can also ask about the store's delivery schedule for any specific fish. There is nothing wrong with asking questions. Every day counts with seafood. If you've ever tasted fish immediately after it was taken from the sea, you know exactly what I mean.

Some fish are farm raised, and some are from the lake or ocean. Don't be afraid to ask which is which. There has been a lot of controversy about pollutants and especially a mercury risk with fish. If you are concerned about this, stick with the *organically* farm-raised fish. Many experts claim that farm raised is much cleaner than ocean or lake fish. Some fish, like shellfish, are bottom feeders (or garbage eaters) and tend to ingest a dirtier diet than other fish. If a bottom-feeding breed is farm raised, like most catfish is today, this is not an issue. Also, ask if any of the fish contain chemicals or preservatives. Some markets do this to increase shelf life, but it's not worth it. Without any preservatives, fish will last a maximum of three days. So buy it and make sure you eat it within that time frame (or else freeze it immediately). Don't settle on unnatural seafood when you don't have to.

When selecting fresh fish, don't select anything that has a strong or unpleasant odor. Fish will have a distinctive smell if it's old. It will also be discolored yellow, brown, or black. Avoid fish with a filmy texture, too. Fish should have a fresh, clean feel to it. If it feels slimy to the touch, this means it has been sitting there a while and it's a little tired now. Fish that has gone bad will have an iodine smell and/or taste. If you happen to buy some bad fish, let your market know. They should be happy to refund your money. Most important, trust your instincts, eyes, fingers, and nose.

With **shrimp** and other types of shellfish, look for a bright white head. That means the shrimp is fresh. When they get old, they get a little yellow or brown. Also, they'll have a slimy feel to them along with an iodine smell.

Clams should be closed 99 percent of the time. If one is slightly open, it could mean that it's dead. It could also mean that it's trying to breathe. To find out, give it a little tap. If nothing happens, it's dead, so don't buy it. If, when you tap it, it quickly closes, you've got a clam that is alive and now a little ticked off. (Again, if you see excessive tapping by another customer, call the Clam Abuse Hotline. I've found them to be even nicer than the folks at Apple Abuse.)

People always ask me which are the best fish to buy. I love fish! I think fish is fantastic, and I eat it often. I love the fact that there are so many varieties. It's not like a choice of just beef or just chicken. **Swordfish, salmon,** and **halibut** are the most popular in the major stores. **Sole** is also popular because it's light and mild tasting. **Escolar** is really in vogue right now. It's been around for a while, but it became really popular last year when President Clinton mentioned that he had it for dinner. Ever since then, its popularity has soared. (Escolar is now as popular as Altoids.)

Salmon is usually available year-round. If I want to avoid the fattiest part of the fish, I just tell my fish guy to cut a piece that doesn't contain a lot of the white lines. This is where the fat is stored. With salmon, it's easy to see because of the white contrast against the pink. The fat, however, will have more flavor. The fattiest part of a salmon is near the head. The leanest part of the fish is near the tail. With humans, it's the opposite. (Unless they're a fathead.) The leanest fish are **red snapper, halibut, mahi mahi,** and **tuna.**

I think my favorite fish is **salmon**. It has so many great qualities. It's really high in calcium, it's got a wonderful flavor, and it's one of the few fish that is really hard to ruin when you cook it. Its flavor is unique. I've had small salmon, really large salmon, and wild salmon, and it always tasted great! I also love **tuna**, especially tuna sashimi (raw tuna). It has a very clean and healthy taste and texture. The Japanese have mastered the art of tuna preparation using soy sauce, sesame, and/or wasabi.

And the last fish that I would put in my top three would be **swordfish**. If you want to feel like you're really eating something hearty, go with swordfish. I love the flavor and dense meatiness of swordfish. In fact, I like to prepare it the same way I *used* to prepare steak, charred on the outside but rare on the inside. It's the perfect meal when you're feeling a little carnivorous.

Chicken

It's important that chicken is free range because not only are the chickens raised on natural grains and allowed to run free (hence, free range), but they are killed in a humane and sanitary way. Select your chicken the same way you select fish. Use your eyes, nose, and fingers. Don't select a chicken with a foul smell, dark discoloration, or slimy texture. The best way to smell for freshness is to smell inside the cavity. Take the bag of giblets out and take a whiff. That's where the smell is strongest. It's perfectly fine to do this at your health food store. (It's just a little embarrassing when one of your friends catches you smelling a chicken's butt!)

Buying the Best Utensils and Cookware

There is an old Australian Aboriginal saying: the more you know, the less you need. Keep this in mind as you shop for your kitchen utensils. It's not necessary that you arm yourself with a designer knife set from Williams Sonoma, but rather with knowledge and experience. Buy the essentials to get started; then add items you need as you gain experience. Don't rush out and buy a bunch of items that will end up wasting valuable kitchen space. Most people get everything they will ever need from their wedding shower. (So, if you got married recently, you're probably all set.) If you're single, don't get married just to get the equipment. (Unless, of course, you register at Williams Sonoma.) If you're a single guy, a decent Swiss

Army knife should do, or maybe just a pizza cutter and some Handi Wipes. Here are the essentials for the rest of us:

Eight-inch chef's knife: This is the knife you will use most. It's an all-purpose knife for chopping, slicing, dicing, and making julienne strips.

Four-inch paring knife: This is the son-of-chef's-knife. This little guy is best for all the jobs that are too small for the chef's knife: some mincing jobs, peeling cucumbers, or cutting out the eyes in a potato (I know that sounds gruesome, especially if you have a thing for Mr. Potato Head).

Eight-inch serrated knife: These are perfect for breads and bagels, but they also work well with fruits like tomatoes. They don't really sharpen well, so you tend to go through these a lot faster than other knives.

Knife sharpener: I like the metal rod type. They're easy to clean and store and often come with knife sets. Sharpen frequently because dull knives are harder to control.

Measuring cups: I recommend a good calibrated set of glass or plastic measuring cups ranging from ¼ cup to 8-cup size. Getting both is not a bad idea. I like to use glass for liquids. Plastic works well with dry ingredients.

Measuring spoons: Get two of the standard sets, which usually include ¼ teaspoon, ½ teaspoon, 1 teaspoon, and 1 tablespoon sizes.

Spatulas: Get a good standard one plus a rubber one for swiping inside bowls, cans, and food processors.

Kitchen scissors: Keep a pair in the kitchen drawer with your other utensils. They come in handy frequently for opening plastic bags, cutting string, and so many other things. You don't want to have to go searching around while you're in the middle of your preparation.

Slotted spoon: This is necessary for removing anything from boiling water.

Tasting spoon: Buy a wooden one so you don't risk burning yourself.

Can opener: Get a top-of-the-line manual one instead of an electric. The electric types are a waste of energy, often get jammed, and are harder to clean.

Colander: This is a necessity. Plastic is better, but stainless steel is okay as long as you don't ever scour it. Wash it gently with a sponge. Once it is scoured, tiny chromium and nickel particles may leach into the food. I recommend the flat-bottom type for stability. They are, however, a little more cumbersome to clean.

Cutting boards: Buy two fairly large boards, one wooden, one polyurethane. (They're relatively inexpensive.) Use the wooden one exclusively for fruits and vegetables, and the polyurethane one for fish and chicken. Because strong smells like garlic and onion can stay with the board and taint your fruit, it may be good to invest in an extra small cutting board as well. When cutting fish and chicken, be sure to scrub the board thoroughly after every use with hot water and a strong soap to avoid salmonella contamination. Wash and dry the wooden board thoroughly after every use as well.

Mandoline: This is certainly not a necessity item, but they're quite inexpensive, starting at about ten dollars, and can really add a lot of excitement to your food preparation. Your vegetables and fruits can be sliced perfectly, evenly, and with style. Be very cautious and follow the directions carefully! The blades on mandolines are very sharp!

Apron: This is a very important item. You immediately realize this on that first day that you get beet juice on your favorite T-shirt. Choose an apron style that makes you feel like a chef: Martha Stewart, Julia Child, or even Bob's Big Boy! It's up to you.

Potholders and oven mitts: Think function, not form, for this one. It's nice to have your potholders match your Early American Settler motif and needlepoint, but the most important criteria are that they grip well and don't burn your hands.

Vegetable steamer: The best kind to get is simple, easy to clean, and designed specifically for steaming. I like the ones with collapsible sides that adjust to any size pot or lid. Avoid aluminum. Stainless steel is okay, but remember not to scour.

Dishcloths: Keep a bunch of clean dishcloths in a drawer ready to go at all times. Also designate a rack to hang the one or two that are in use.

Plastic freezer and sandwich bags: These are indispensable for practically anything you can think of: freezing, storing, separating, organizing toiletries for traveling, everything.

Plastic wrap: For sealing leftovers in bowls and covering some dishes before microwaving.

Small paper bags: For ripening tomatoes and avocados, steaming peppers, and so on.

Well, that was fun. I hope this information helps you so that the next time you're in a health food store, you won't feel so lost. And if you're an old pro, it never hurts to review the basics.

4

Healthy Conversions

So many people are fearful about starting a new and healthier way of living and eating because they are so afraid they will have to give up the things they love most. They say things like, "I love meat loaf!" And "I still need my cookies and milk." "I don't want to give up all my favorite comfort foods and my mom's best recipes from my childhood." Or "I'll never be able to taste pastrami or bake an apple pie again."

But don't worry. You won't have to give up any of the things you love, because *everything* is convertible! You just have to know *how* to convert and *what* to convert it to. It's really very simple. We're going to provide you with charts to help you, in addition to tips and suggestions to guide you while you're shopping and cooking. In place of sugar, you will learn how to use sugar substitutes such as honey, date sugar, or barley malt, depending on the recipe, situation, and your personal taste. For dairy products, you can use soy, rice, or nut products. You will see that even meats and lunchmeats have marvelous vegan substitutes with great flavors and textures. Ideally, you should use tofu and soy products, but if you are still eating chicken and turkey, you can make turkey meat loaf instead of using beef.

The world of soy opened up to me twenty-one years ago. Since then, I have learned that I can eat everything I have always loved, and will be able to for the rest of my life. The progress in the soy industry in those twenty-one years is amazing. When I first started, there was no such thing as soy cheese, much less soy bacon, soy pastrami, and soy ground round. Now, however, there are so many varieties that it's easy to find one that you really like. One of my favorite flavors as a child was pork sausage. I loved Sunday mornings. It was the only day of the week that my father would cook breakfast. He always made Polish eggs and pork sausage. (He was Polish and he liked to make scrambled eggs with milk in a pan. Therefore, Polish eggs.) I will forever associate the smell of sizzling sausage with those special Sunday mornings.

Now, instead of pork sausage, I eat soy sausage. It still gives me that warm cozy Sunday morning feeling because it smells the same, only it's healthier and cleaner. I especially love Yves and Soy Boy. I use soy sausage in every recipe that I would have put regular sausage in, including Thanksgiving stuffing.

Remember, you can *always* convert your favorite recipe to a healthier one. The products are available. You just have to know how to change one to the other. Be careful that you don't substitute one bad food for another bad food. Some substitution options are better than others. Study the conversion charts carefully so you can make selections that suit your needs and tastes. It will help you understand, for example, differences in sweetness levels: one tablespoon of sugar might equal one tablespoon of Sucanat, but equals only three-quarters of a tablespoon of honey.

Also, as your palate becomes cleaner and you can better appreciate subtler flavors, continue to try different substitutes. You might discover that you actually prefer the hearty flavor of date sugar over the sickeningly sweet flavor of sugar. Over time you will realize that food doesn't have to kill you to taste good.

The main substitutes to focus on should be sugar, dairy, and meat. The best way to illustrate this is to use a few examples that are typical American staples: macaroni and cheese, meat loaf, chocolate chip cookies, brownies, and chili. Compare the ingredients used in typical recipes and in our converted healthy ones.

As you can see, many of the ingredients we are used to seeing in a classic recipe can be converted to a healthier Total Health Makeover (THM) version. The following charts will give you some guidelines for converting your favorite recipes.

CLASSIC MACARONI AND CHEESE

MAKES 4 TO 6 SERVINGS

Cooked macaroni (8 ounces dry)
2 eggs, beaten
3 cups milk
2 tablespoons butter, cut in pieces
1¼ cups cubed sharp cheese
1 teaspoon salt

THM MACARONI AND CHEESE

MAKES 4 TO 6 SERVINGS

Cooked wheatless elbow pasta (12 ounces dry)
1 package Mori-Nu firm tofu
¼ cup plain soy milk
1 pat soy butter (optional)
1 brick mild cheddar soy cheese, grated

CLASSIC MEAT LOAF

MAKES 6 TO 8 SERVINGS

2 pounds ground beef
3 slices white bread, broken in pieces
1 cup milk
1 egg
1 tablespoon Worcestershire sauce
¼ onion, minced
1¼ teaspoons salt

THM MEAT LOAF

MAKES 6 TO 8 SERVINGS

2 pounds Gimme Lean
2 slices wheat bread
1 teaspoon olive oil
1½ cups soy milk
2 large eggs, lightly beaten
3 tablespoons Dijon mustard
1 small Spanish onion, chopped
2 to 3 cloves garlic, finely chopped
1 teaspoon dried oregano
1 teaspoon black pepper
½ cup chopped fresh parsley
¾ cup ketchup or barbecue sauce

CLASSIC CHOCOLATE CHIP COOKIES

MAKES ABOUT 5 DOZEN COOKIES

1 cup butter, softened
¾ cup granulated sugar
¾ cup packed light brown sugar
1 teaspoon vanilla extract
2 eggs
2¼ cups all-purpose flour
1 teaspoon baking soda
½ teaspoon salt
One 11.5-ounce package choco-
    late chips

THM CHOCOLATE CHIP COOKIES

MAKES 8 DOZEN 2-INCH COOKIES

1 cup soy margarine
1 cup Sucanat
½ cup date sugar
1 teaspoon vanilla extract
2 large eggs
2½ cups unsifted all-purpose
    flour
1 level teaspoon baking soda
1 level teaspoon salt
One 12-ounce package semi-
    sweet non-dairy chocolate
    chips (such as Tropical
    Source)

CLASSIC BROWNIES

MAKES 16 BROWNIES

4 ounces unsweetened choco-
    late
1 cup (2 sticks) butter
1¾ cups sugar
4 large eggs
1 tablespoon vanilla extract
1 cup all-purpose flour
½ teaspoon salt
Walnuts (optional)

THM BROWNIES

MAKES 16 BROWNIES

4 ounces unsweetened choco-
    late
1 cup (2 sticks) soy margarine
1¾ cups Sucanat or maple sugar
4 large eggs
1 tablespoon vanilla extract
1 cup unbleached all-purpose
    flour
½ teaspoon salt
Walnuts (optional)

CLASSIC CHILI

MAKES ABOUT 8 CUPS

1 teaspoon olive oil
1 medium Spanish onion,
  chopped
4 cloves garlic, chopped or
  pressed
1 pound ground beef
1 to 3 tablespoons chili powder
2 tablespoons dried oregano
1 teaspoon ground cumin
1 teaspoon ground cinnamon
1 cup beef stock
One 28-ounce can crushed
  tomatoes
Two 16-ounce cans dark red
  kidney beans, drained and
  rinsed
Salt and pepper to taste

THM CHILI

MAKES ABOUT 8 CUPS

1 teaspoon olive oil
1 medium Spanish onion,
  chopped
4 cloves garlic, chopped or
  pressed
1 pound soy meat
1 to 3 tablespoons chili powder
2 tablespoons dried oregano
1 teaspoon ground cumin
1 teaspoon ground cinnamin
1 cup veggie stock
One 28-ounce can crushed
  tomatoes
Two 16-ounce cans dark red
  kidney beans, drained and
  rinsed
2 tablespoons Bragg Liquid
  Aminos
Salt and pepper to taste

SWEETENER CONVERSION CHART

Sweetener	Source/Taste	Form	Relative Sweetness
White sugar	Pure sweetness. Highly refined from sugar cane.	Granulated	1
Brown sugar	White sugar with a dye job. Slight molasses taste	Granulated	1
Fructose	From corn. Very sweet.	Granulated	2
Honey	Extracted from flower nectar by bees. It's 20 to 60 percent sweeter than sugar, so use less.	Honeycomb, thick liquid, or cream	1.3
Maple syrup	Drawn from sap of maple trees. Use only pure U.S. organic syrup to avoid formaldehyde and additives.	Syrup	0.6
Maple sugar	Dehydrated maple syrup.	Granulated	0.6
Barley malt	Sprouted barley. Strong distinctive flavor (like molasses).	Dark liquid	0.6
Brown rice syrup	Brown rice and various enzymes. Mild butterscotch flavor.	Thick liquid	0.7
Fruit juice concentrate	Peach, pear, grape, pineapple are most common.	Syrup or liquid	1.3
Molasses	Light and Barbados have lighter molasses taste than sorghum or blackstrap.	Syrup	0.6
Date sugar	Ground, dehydrated dates	Granulated	0.6
Sucanat or Rapadura	Organic evaporated cane juice. Minerals and molasses are retained.	Granulated	1
Stevia	A perennial shrub of the aster family	Whole or broken leaves, coarse ground, powder extract, or liquid extract	8 to 300 times, depending on quality and whether it is leaf or extract

Substitution for 1 Cup Sugar	Reduction of Total Liquid	Additional Comments
		May not be vegetarian. Beef bone used in some refineries. (Not recommended.)
		Same as white sugar. (Not recommended.)
		Highly refined. Sweetness unstable. (Not recommended.)
⅔ to ¾ cup	⅛ to ¼ cup. Add ¼ teaspoon of baking soda per cup honey.	Reduce oven 25 degrees and adjust the baking time.
¾ to 1 cup	⅛ to ¼ cup. Add ¼ teaspoon baking soda per cup maple syrup.	Use in all baked goods. The moisture retention makes it especially good in cakes.
1 cup	No reduction of liquid. Add ⅛ teaspoon baking soda per cup maple sugar.	Use in all baked goods. Store in airtight container and sift before using.
1⅓ to 1½ cups	¼ cup. Add ¼ teaspoon baking soda per cup barley malt.	Stay away from barley/corn malt syrup. Buy only 100 percent barley malt. Organic available.
1⅓ cups to 1½ cups	¼ cup per cup brown rice syrup. ¼ teaspoon baking soda per cup brown rice syrup.	Baked goods with brown rice syrup tend to be hard or very crisp. Combine with another sweetener such as maple for cakes.
⅔ cup	⅓ cup per cup of fruit sweetener. Add ¼ teaspoon baking soda per cup fruit juice concentrate.	Reduce oven 25 degrees. Store in refrigerator but use at room temperature.
½ cup		Good in corn muffins, rye bread, gingerbread, and cookies
1 cup		Add hot water to dissolve date sugars before using. Use in crisps, crunches, as sprinkle or topping. Purchase date sugar made from unsulfured, organically grown dates.
1 cup		Sift prior to using.
1 teaspoon	Experiment in converting recipes, adjusting liquid and dry ingredients to make up for lack of bulk.	May soon be in easier form to use. Significantly enhances the flavor and nutritional value of food.

HEALTHY SUBSTITUTIONS

In Place of	Substitute
Baking powder and soda	Use health food store brand only.
Butter	Soy margarine (Earth Balance)
Chocolate	Non-sugar non-dairy chocolate chips (Tropical Source)
Cornstarch (for thickening)	Arrowroot (when using arrowroot as a substitute for flour thickening or cornstarch, reduce the amount by one half)
2 tablespoons butter mixed with 1 tablespoon flour to thicken soups and sauces (7 grams fat)	2 tablespoons kuzu (0 grams fat)
Eggs	Egg whites (1 egg = 2 egg whites *or* 2 eggs = 3 egg whites)
Mayonnaise (1 tablespoon = 11 grams fat)	Tofu mayonnaise (1 tablespoon = 3.5 grams fat)
Meat	Beans (especially soybeans), grains, nuts
Salt	Kelp granules, garlic (fresh or powdered), and herbs
Vinegar	Use only pure apple cider vinegar or fresh lemon juice.
White flour	Whole-grain flours (for baking, use 100 percent

	whole-grain pastry flours). When substituting whole-grain flour for white flour in a recipe, use approximately 20 percent more moisture because of the greater absorption of the whole-wheat flour due to the presence of bran and wheat germ. Also, use about 10 percent less shortening.
Cow's milk	Rice milk, soybean milk, nut milks (coconut milk, almond milk, etc.)
1 cup milk	1 cup rice or soy milk or other milk substitute *or* ½ cup milk substitute and ½ cup water *or* ½ cup juice and ½ cup water *or* 1 cup water
1 cup milk (for baking)	1 cup rice or soy milk or other milk substitute *or* 1 cup water and 2 tablespoons soy *or* rice margarine
1 cup buttermilk	½ cup milk substitute, ½ cup water, and 1 tablespoon vinegar or lemon juice
Light cream	Silk plain soy milk
Heavy cream	Silk plain soy cream
Sour cream	Soy sour cream
Cream cheese	Nayonaise or soy cream cheese

5

Preparation, Cooking, and Presentation Methods

Cleaning Fruits and Vegetables

It's important that you clean all of your fruits and vegetables. Try using a little bit of Dr. Bronner's Soap diluted in water. It's very mild and tasteless, so it will not interfere with the flavor of the food. Let your fruits and vegetables soak for a couple of minutes, then wash them off. To remove bugs from organic fruits and vegetables, soak them in a mild solution of vinegar and water (ten parts water, one part vinegar). The bugs will float to the top. (A great tip from the produce man at Whole Foods Market in Los Angeles.)

Cutting Fruits and Vegetables

When cutting fruits and vegetables, it is best that you work with quality knives and sharpen them frequently. Quality knives are easier and safer to work with and will last much longer, making them a better buy in the long run. Sharpen them frequently, because a dull knife requires more uncontrolled and therefore more dangerous force. As you are chopping, focus on the task at hand. Cuts are usually the result of carelessness and/or external distractions. The deepest I ever cut myself was when I was working as a waitress and sliced into a bagel while I was talking to someone. I learned two lessons: always pay attention and *never* cut a bagel while it's in your hand. It's best if you secure the fruit or vegetable on the cutting surface with your knuckles tucked in tightly so that only knuckles, and *not* fingertips, are touching the vegetable. (If you're a baseball fan, think of the grip used for throwing a knuckleball.) This is another precaution to avoid cuts. Remember: most of these dishes are intended to be vegetarian. "Stir-fried knuckles" no longer qualifies as vegan.

Chopping Fruits and Vegetables

When chopping fruits and vegetables, use a wooden chopping board as opposed to a marble one. Marble will blunt your knives. It's important to create a flat surface on the vegetable you're cutting so that it has stability. After your first cut, place that flat side down. If you're going to cut the vegetable into julienne strips or cubes, it's a good idea to square it off first: cutting off the round surface on all four sides so that you now have one large cube to work with.

- Julienne: Cut into ¼- to ½-inch-thick by 2-inch-long strips. Think of the strips in a Julienne (chef's) salad.

- Cube: Take the julienne cut a step further and cut uniform pieces of ½- to 1-inch cubes.
- Dice: Smaller version of cube. Cut your cubes ⅛- to ¼-inch size.
- Mince: This refers to cutting into the tiniest uneven pieces.
- Slicing: Slice about ½ inch thick at approximately a forty-five-degree angle.

Methods of Cooking

There are three different types of cooking methods: dry heat, moist heat, and a combination of the two. Dry heat methods use hot air or oil to cook. This includes broiling, grilling, roasting, baking, sautéing, stir-frying, and deep-frying. Moist heat cooking includes boiling, poaching, blanching, simmering, and steaming. Stewing would fall into the category of the combination method.

Boiling

It's usually better to poach or blanch vegetables than to boil them. Boiling, which is cooking food by keeping it submerged in a boiling liquid for an extended period of time, removes many of the nutrients. Boiling is more appropriate for cooking starches like potatoes, pastas, and rice. With boiling, it's important that you have enough liquid and that it is already boiling when you add the food. An insufficient amount of liquid will take too long to return to its boiling point and the food will not cook properly. The rice and pasta, for example, will turn out too sticky. For most preparations using the boiling method, keep the following in mind:

- Bring a sufficient amount of water to a boil.
- Add the rice, pasta, or whatever you're cooking to the boiling water and stir gently.
- Let the water return to a boil.
- Continue boiling while stirring occasionally until food is cooked to desired consistency.
- Drain the water in a colander.
- Transfer to a hot, or at least warm, bowl or dish.

Poaching and Simmering

Poaching is cooking by submerging a food in a liquid that is slightly cooler than simmering (as opposed to a boiling liquid). Poaching is much better than boiling as a way of preserving nutrients in vegetables.

- Prepare the item by cutting to appropriate size and/or trimming the excess fat.
- Allow the liquid, preferably seasoned, to come to a simmer (use slightly less heat for poaching). Make sure there is enough water to submerge the food completely.
- Slowly lower the food into the simmering liquid. If the food being cooked is very delicate, use a wire mesh or wire rack to hold it together. An open serving spoon is also useful for lowering the food.
- Keep the temperature constant as you proceed. Never allow the liquid to boil.
- When the food is done, transfer it to a hot or warm serving plate.
- Add extra seasoning or some of the liquid back if you like.

If you are poaching a salmon, it is a good idea to save the water. You can always use the salmon-flavored water to add flavor to a vegetable side dish or add it back to the salmon if it comes out a little dry.

Blanching

Blanching is cooking, or partially cooking, by briefly submerging a food in a boiling liquid. Blanching, like poaching, is a better method of cooking vegetables than boiling.

- Have your food prepared to be submerged (i.e., beans cut and rinsed, broccoli in the size you want to serve, and so on).
- Blanch vegetables quickly in boiling water to avoid oxidation.

Steaming

Steaming is best of all for most vegetables. This gentle way of cooking retains both flavor and nutrients. With steaming, the food is suspended above and never actually touches the boiling water. Steaming works best when you use a steamer, which is specifically designed for steaming. If you don't own a steamer, you can suspend a mesh pot, or something similar, over a pot of boiling water. My advice is to invest in a steamer. It's worth it. The basic method for steaming is as follows:

- Bring the liquid in the bottom container to a full boil.
- Cover the steamer to allow it to heat fully.
- Remove the lid to add the food to the top compartment. (Be cautious. The steam is 212 degrees Fahrenheit or more.) Then replace the lid.
- Lower the heat to bring the liquid down to just a simmer.
- Continue until food is cooked as you desire.
- Transfer food to a hot or warm serving bowl or dish.

With vegetables, always err on the side of undercooking. Slightly undercooked vegetables have the most flavor and texture. When you're steaming a vegetable, try seasoning the water in the bottom pan of the steamer with vegetable bouillon. The natural flavors of the vegetable itself will be enhanced as it absorbs the bouillon essence. This is perfect for those of you who steam broccoli and then add too much salt at the table because you feel the steamed broccoli lacks flavor. Another option is to pour the bouillon broth over the steamed vegetable afterward as a coating. (This makes the vegetable so tasty!) Steamed spinach is especially good with a bouillon cube in the bottom. If your spouse or children still resist the idea of eating steamed vegetables, you can top it off with Bragg Liquid Aminos and drizzled soy margarine. (My kids love vegetables this way!) You can also try adding other flavors to the boiling water in your steamer, such as herbs, lemon, or wine. (Of course, don't use wine for steaming dishes you will be serving to your kids.)

Broiling and Grilling

Broil when you want fish to be crispy outside but moist inside. This works especially well for fish that has been coated with something like nuts or crumbs. Broiling tends to sear the outside while leaving the inside moist and tender, whereas baking tends to cook the whole fish evenly.

People often lump broiling and grilling in the same category. Both use radiant heat; however, the basic difference is that with broiling, the fire, or heat source, is above the food; with grilling, the fire is below the food. If you don't have a grill at home and a recipe that calls for grilling, feel free to broil instead. Here are some basic guidelines for grilling and broiling.

- Prepare the food by slicing and seasoning as stated in the recipe.
- Preheat the broiler or grill to the temperature recommended in the recipe.
- Place the food on the grill for a part of the time, then change the angle to give the food a grilled and/or broiled crisscross pattern.
- Repeat this on the other side after flipping the food over.

Baking and Roasting

The methods of baking and roasting are basically the same. The difference comes from *what* you're cooking, not *how* you're cooking. Foods you associate with a bakery (breads, pastries, and other sweet baked goods) are baked, while roasting is associated more with meats and vegetables. I use a great product for baking and roasting called Baker's Magic. It's a soy margarine and flour spray for your pans. You just spray your pans with it before cooking to keep food from sticking. It's excellent!

- Prepare food to be cooked by salting, seasoning, mixing, or shaping, depending on what you're making.
- Preheat the oven, usually between 275 and 425 degrees, depending on what the recipe calls for.
- Remove the item when it is done and allow it to sit and cool for a few minutes before serving.

Sautéing and Stir-Frying

A wok is perfectly designed for stir-frying. You automatically use less oil since it mixes evenly with the food at the bottom of the wok. A wok is great, but not a necessity. Use oil as sparingly as possible. Pretend it costs five hundred dollars a bottle (some of those new designer oils almost do). The vegetables themselves will yield plenty of water, creating a great base for sautéing (especially vegetables like mushrooms). You will find that you really won't need much oil. You can actually sauté mushrooms in nothing but a few herbs and/or salt and pepper for flavoring if you need it.

When you stir-fry, try different flavored oils that will change the flavor of the food. There are so many different oils now like hazelnut, walnut, hot pepper, porcini, white truffle, black truffle, and on and on. They all vary in viscosity (e.g., white truffle oil will be much heavier than hazelnut oil). If, for example, you're making a chicken-almond stir-fry and the recipe calls for peanut oil, don't be afraid to experiment with something like almond oil or sesame oil. You might be pleasantly surprised. Don't let yourself be a boring cook and use the same safflower or canola oil for every vegetable dish. Instead, try oil with some flavor that could bring a simple dish to life, like olive oil infused with basil, rosemary, or hot chili peppers.

One thing nice about stir-frying is that it's a great way to clean out your refrigerator when you've got vegetables that are near their final days and you don't want them to go to waste. It's the kind of cooking opportunity that lends itself to walking in at 6:00 P.M. from a long day at work, taking whatever happens to be in your refrigerator at the time, and making a fantastic stir-fry! Anything and everything might work well together. Making soup is another option for your vegetables on death row. (And you thought you had nothing in your refrigerator.)

- Prepare food to be cooked by seasoning and cutting into small strips. Try to make the strips uniform so they'll cook somewhat evenly.
- Place the wok or pan over the flame and allow it to heat up a bit.
- Add a very small amount of oil and let it heat up but not smoke.
- Cook each food in the order of its cooking time, starting with the heaviest and driest (i.e., celery or carrots before tomatoes or mushrooms).
- Place the food in the pan and continually move the food around by flipping and shaking the pan and/or by stirring with a utensil. Do this until the food is cooked the way you like it.

The essence of stir-frying is that the food is cooked quickly over high heat with very little oil.

Deep-Frying

In deep-frying the food is entirely submerged in oil. Foods that are deep-fried are usually breaded or battered first. The best advice I can give about deep-frying is DON'T DO IT! It's the most fattening and least healthy method of cooking. It's also a turnoff once you have a clean palate.

IDEAL USES FOR NATURAL OILS

Oil	Taste and Properties	Culinary Uses
Almond	Strong, toasted nut; low smoke point	Excellent in salad dressings or chicken salad, drizzled over fish, or in nut-flavored baked goods; not suitable for deep-frying
Avocado	Rich, warm; high smoke point	Excellent in salads, on pasta; suitable for fast-frying, sautéing, and deep-frying
Canola	Light, clear, bland; high smoke point; all-purpose	Blends well for mayonnaise and dressings; especially good for baking
Corn	Pleasant "corny" flavor; general use	Good for baking (especially pie crusts), cooking, and making popcorn
Olive	Distinctive, fruity; all-purpose	Good for frying, sautéing, salad dressings, pasta sauces, some baking; not suitable for deep-frying
Peanut	Slightly heavy, nutty; may "flash" at high temperature	Excellent in Oriental stir-fries, Thai and Indonesian dishes; also good for salads
Safflower	Fairly bland; good for frying since it does not foam; general use	Good for frying, sautéing, salad dressings, baking; use to dilute stronger oils and in mayonnaise
Sesame	Toasted sesame has a rich, strong flavor, while untoasted is lighter, more bland	Use toasted in salad dressings, Oriental dishes; untoasted for stir-fries
Soy	Bold if unrefined; high smoke point; general use	Used commercially in margarine and mayonnaise
Sunflower	Nearly tasteless and odorless; all-purpose	Good in salad dressings, stir-fries, mayonnaise; use for frying, sautéing, and to dilute stronger oils
Walnut	Silky, rich, mildly nutty; low smoke point	Excellent for sautéing and in salad dressings, pasta, potato and chicken salads

THE BEST OILS FOR VARIOUS COOKING METHODS

Method	Temperature	Best Oils
Frying	High heat (up to 500 degrees)	Avocado, apricot kernel, rice bran, sesame, peanut, high oleic safflower, sunflower
Baking, sautéing, sauces	Medium heat (up to 375 degrees)	Canola, corn, grape seed, safflower, sunflower, soy, walnut, sesame
Light sautéing, pressure cooking, soups	Moderate heat (up to 320 degrees)	Corn, grape seed, olive, peanut, pumpkin, safflower, sesame, soy, walnut

Presentation of Food—a.k.a. Razzle Dazzle 'Em!

So many people think that health food is boring and ugly. They probably saw too many dishes overflowing with sprouts in the sixties and seventies. Food doesn't have to kill you to taste good, and food doesn't have to be ugly to make you feel better. Most of you already understand this, but what about those nights when you throw a dinner party for your baby-back-rib-eatin' supervisor and his cream-puff-pastry-lovin' wife? How do you prepare something that is healthy and still looks appetizing for *them*?

I believe that the answer is not to try and fake your guests into thinking that that they're eating their usual junk food. You'll never make tofu with scallions look like a bacon cheeseburger. Instead, showcase the subtle, natural beauty of the healthy food you're serving.

Approach this like an artist. Play with different types of garnish. If you really want to get into this, try growing your own herbs and garnishes. It's easy. Herbs are essentially weeds, so you can stick them almost anywhere and practically neglect them. They do well without much water or with too much sun. You can abuse them and they'll still be there in the morning. They're like a boyfriend who won't take a hint. Also, home-grown herbs are usually more beautiful than what you buy in the store, and it's fun to say things to your guests like, "Oh, the parsley? Yes, isn't it beautiful! I grow it on my patio."

Along with garnish arrangement, focus on the central ingredient in the dish you're serving. Try to use that to tell a story about the dish. For example, if you're serving watercress soup, just drop one of the prettier sprigs of watercress on top so your guests know that the soup is green because of watercress and not basil or broccoli. Do the same thing with carrot soup or cake. Drop a thinly sliced carrot curl with the end piece cut at a forty-five-degree angle like a ribbon. This works well with things like chives, too. Use the natural beauty of the vegetable. Carefully study the pattern in which it grows in nature and honor that in your cut and presentation.

Try copying from books a little bit at first to get a feel for this. Then experiment on your own. It can really be rewarding when your culinary and artistic abilities come together.

Kitchen Tips

1. Keep steel wool from rusting by wrapping aluminum foil around it and leaving it in the freezer.
2. To make measuring dry products less messy, fold a piece of wax paper, open it up, and measure over the paper. Pour the remainder back into its original container.
3. Avoid tomato or dark stains on plastic containers by spraying with no-stick cooking spray before filling.
4. If you don't have a salad spinner, try drying lettuce with a blow dryer. Or you can wrap the lettuce in a dish towel, grab the ends, and let your arm whirl like a helicopter.
5. Make weighing chopped foods easier by weighing them in coffee filters.
6. Keep vegetables fresher by lining the bottom of the vegetable bin with a paper towel. It absorbs the excess moisture.
7. If cork ends up inside the wine bottle, use a coffee filter to strain the wine.
8. Dry the inside of rubber gloves with a blow dryer.
9. Keep garbage bags from slipping by wrapping an old panty-hose waistline around the top.
10. Plastic scouring pads are better for pots and pans. Rinse and soak your pots as soon as you're done cooking. This will make them easier to clean and will prevent tiny particles from coming loose from the surfaces.

6

What You Will or Will Not Find in These Recipes

The Current Trend of High-Protein, Low-Carbohydrate (High-Fat!) Diets

One of the most common questions I've been asked during my recent book tour and on my website is how I feel about the current "resuscitation" of the many versions of the high-protein, low-carbohydrate (and therefore high-fat) diets that were popular back in the sixties and seventies. My answer is this: these diets, which stress the meticulous counting and restriction of carbohydrates while promoting high protein (with its high fat), are the same types of diets I tried when I was a teenager. It took me years to undo the damage it caused my stomach and metabolism.

At that time, my sister Christal and I decided that we would go on diets together. It was a little experiment to see which of two popular yet different diets would work better. I decided to follow the one that counted calories, and she chose the high-protein diet that severely limited carbohydrates. After a week, she was losing more weight than I was, so I decided to switch to her diet. But after only ten days, I became severely carbohydrate-starved. All that protein made me ravenous for carbohydrates. I remember that I ate an entire chocolate frosted Sara Lee cake in three bites. (And I don't even like chocolate!) I started to put the weight back on. Within a month, I gained it *all* back and then some. Determined, I tried this diet the next month, resolving not to fall off the wagon after ten days. But sure enough, in time I felt the same deprivation. And while I didn't binge out on carbs, even eating the few graham crackers or piece of toast I craved made me gain weight. My body just didn't know how to handle even a few carbohydrates. With this high-protein, low-carbohydrate, high-fat diet, I not only gained back all of my weight, but my skin broke out and I had bad breath. I also became dehydrated, constipated, and had to pee all the time because my kidneys were not functioning properly. My body was completely out of balance. Christal had the same reaction. Needless to say, our date books were empty the weeks we were on this diet. We did, however, have each other to console on those lonely Saturday nights while we ate our pork rinds.

So, even back then, when I was trying every diet imaginable, I learned that this ridiculous and gimmicky high-protein, low-carbohydrate, high-fat diet was unhealthy and harmful in the long run. And even though I tried it again years later (I tried *every* diet at least three times before I discovered the Total Health Makeover), I had the same reaction. After about two weeks, I would feel out of balance again with dehydration, constipation, bad skin, and bad breath, *and* I would regain the weight.

After twenty years of experimenting with hundreds of diets while carefully studying the human body, I have learned that the amount of protein and fat that people consume with this type of fad diet is dangerous to both our digestive and cardiovascular systems. Our intestinal tract is not designed for the amount of protein you end up consuming on this diet. The twists and turns in our very long and complicated intestinal tract are typical of other vegetarian animals. Observe the animals in the wild that have the closest DNA makeup to that of humans—chimpanzees, orangutans, and gorillas. (I don't mean you should actually hang out with them like Jane Goodall. Just read about them on the Internet.) You will find that their diet consists mainly of fruits, leaves, vegetables, and insects (you're going to love my caterpillar salad on page 184. Don't get nervous—I'm only kidding.)

This does, however, reveal that *some* animal protein is normal. Animal protein makes up about 3 percent of their diet. Having animal protein for *most* meals is very risky. I think it's funny that we are the most intelligent of all animals, yet other animals, left to their own instincts, will pick better food for themselves and have less disease and much less obesity than we do. As smart as we are, we humans continue to eat bad foods like white flour, refined sugar, red meat, and breast milk from a cow. We even feed this junk to our children. Every day our kids get filled up at school with something meaty, cheesy, creamy, or sugary, full of chemicals and devoid of life. It's always something that's not real; it's something bought in a typical grocery store just for the convenience of it. Dead, fat laden, chemical food is served to children every day in school. And then later on we wonder why they have diseases, addictions, and obesity as adults. Kids instead should learn good nutritional habits and about healthy food that is also tasty. We should train their palates to enjoy good, healthy, *real* foods.

I can only think of the high-protein, low-carbohydrate, high-fat way of eating as population control. The amount of heart disease and colon cancer that we are going to develop by making this diet a fad again is a way to keep the population down. The number of people who will get sick and eventually die as a result of the colon blocking, artery clogging, and cardiovascular distress brought on by this way of eating will keep the population at a nice manageable number. With all of the good information that we now have about what people should be eating (fruits, vegetables, whole grains, legumes, lean proteins), can you think of it as anything else? Making meat more than 30 percent of our diet is suicide.

I get upset when somebody tells me that they are not allowed to have a good healthy bowl of cholesterol-lowering oatmeal, but instead will eat a heart- and colon-clogging cheese omelet with bacon because it's *allowed* on their "protein" diet. I can spot a person on a high-protein, low-carbohydrate, high-fat diet in a second. Along with a drawn-out, sallow look on their face, they usually have those telltale big, dark circles under their eyes because their kidneys are so overworked. One of the other signs is that their breath is bad. A person will have bad breath on this diet not only because of all the animal protein they are consuming, but also because their body is in a state of ketosis. They often look thinner at first, but then a yo-yo pattern develops.

I recently saw a friend who had lost thirty-five pounds on this diet, and then I saw her again after she gained forty-five pounds back. She had regained the thirty-five *plus* ten more! I've seen this happen again and again because the human body has evolved into one that is designed to eat plant foods: complex carbohydrates, fruits, and vegetables. Look at our teeth. We don't have a mouth full of sharp incisor teeth like a flesh-eating animal has. We have molars to grind and break the grain. We don't sweat through our tongues like a flesh-eating animal does. (I don't care how hot it gets where you live.) A flesh-eating animal has a short intestinal tract and a large stomach. We have a long (twenty-seven feet!) intestinal tract and a small stomach by comparison. The unnatural stress that a flesh-eating, high-protein, low-carbohydrate, high-fat diet puts on the human body causes it to malfunction. I'm not saying you should avoid protein. I'm only saying that your protein should come primarily from the healthier sources: beans (especially soy), nuts, grains, and fish.

There is no balance to a diet that wipes out an important food group like complex carbohydrates. Each food group contributes to the body in a different but equally important way. You really cannot eliminate a food group without negative consequences. People often say to me "What about your program? You eliminate dairy products. That's one of the food groups." And I always say to them, "It's only a food group if you're a baby calf." (Besides, the contribution dairy products make to the body can be obtained in healthier ways through soy and other plant sources.)

The Benefits of Food Combining

One of the reasons carbohydrates have a bad reputation is that people usually eat them in *combination* with proteins. In fact, it is America's most common dietary mix: meat and potatoes, pizza, burgers and sandwiches. Avoiding this "mix" is the underlying premise behind food combining. Proteins and starches require different digestive enzymes, which function at different pH levels in the body. Pepsin digests protein in the highly acidic environment of the stomach, and starches prefer the alkaline environment of the intestines. Combining these two types of food traps them and slows down the digestive process. The undigested food causes digestive problems such as gas, bloating, and constipation, as well as weight gain.

Along with the bad rap that carbohydrates get from being eaten with proteins is the fact that the carbohydrates that most people eat are refined and processed with excess sugar and salt. Protein diet enthusiasts love to capitalize on all this carb negativity by unfairly lumping the bad carbohydrates (white-flour carbs like bagels, cakes, cookies, and pies) together with the good complex carbohydrates (whole-grain carbs like brown rice, oatmeal, and couscous). They might all be under the carbohydrate category but they're *not* the same. Your body doesn't break them down or utilize them in the same way.

Whole Grains vs. Refined

A whole grain has three parts: the bran, the germ, and the endosperm. When grain is refined, the bran and the germ are removed, leaving only the inside core, the endosperm. The bran, which is the outer shell, contains B vitamins, phosphorus, potassium, and most important, a high concentration of the fiber that is necessary to carry the other parts of the whole grain through the digestive tract. Without this, the digestion process is less efficient. During refining, this extremely important component of this nearly perfect food is removed along with the middle layer, the germ, which contains protein, complex carbohydrates, unsaturated fats, B-complex vitamins, vitamin E, and iron. All of those rich vitamins, minerals, and that necessary digestion-helping fiber become waste product at the refining plant. It's very sad. All of that intestinal-scrubbing fiber ends up in the factory garbage can. Perhaps the scrubbing fiber prefers that fate to . . . you know . . . the "alternative" location, but the lack of these little helpers is not good for you . . . or your colon.

High-protein, low-carbohydrate, high-fat diets claim that all carbohydrates raise your insulin level and that is what makes you crave more and more carbohydrates until it feels like an addiction. But it is the *sugar* in processed carbohydrates that people usually become addicted to. The most commonly eaten carbohydrates have sugar in them: pastries, cakes, cookies, and all that other bad stuff you should avoid. Yet these diets lump these carbohydrates together with whole grains. You won't have a problem if you keep the white refined flours and white sugar out of your carbohydrate consumption. It's the overprocessed, overrefined white flours that bulk you up. It's the sugar that ferments and slows down your digestion.

There is no way you are going to live permanently on a high-protein, low-carbohydrate, high-fat diet. Not only will you desperately crave carbs, your body will "dry up inside" because your kidneys are so overworked. It is as if your body is always draining itself.

I can't tell you how many people on high-protein, low-carbohydrate, high-fat diets tell me things like "I'm losing some weight, but I'm so constipated!" or "I don't know if I can take one more glass of water!" These diets require a large quantity of water because eating all of that protein is so dehydrating. Unfortunately, drinking all that water dilutes the digestive juices that are so necessary to break down all that protein. It's a vicious cycle.

People ask me why high-protein, high-fat diets are so successful if they're so bad for you. It's because these diets tell people exactly what they want to hear: you can eat all the foods that are bad for you and still lose weight. People would rather be thin than healthy. (I know, I was one of them.) But I'm excited to tell you that you can be thin and healthy. You can be the animal you were meant to be. You can be the best version of yourself.

At first, these high-protein diets are a big hit and gain a lot of momentum. Then people get wise to them and their creators have to hide for several years until the public forgets. That's about when these diets make their comeback. It's like those money pyramids and chain letters. At first they seem like a great way to make money, so people join. Then people realize what a scam it is, and the scam artists are forced to go underground and wait for the public to forget again.

Food is like fashion. Fashion trends have to constantly change for the fashion industry to make a profit. After the hemlines go up, it's not long before they have to come down again to encourage people to buy a newer product. Fashion has to keep changing. It's the same with the diet industry. This particular high-protein, low-carbohydrate, high-fat diet was first fashionable in the late sixties and then again in the seventies. It has only come back because it sold books back then and everyone has forgotten by now about the bad side effects. Most people do not want to face the fact that you need to stick with *all* of the food groups. You need to exercise and stay away from fatty meats and dairy products. Simply put, you should stay away from something that's not meant for human consumption. Focus more on the quality of what you eat and not so much on the quantity. Time and time again I've seen that if you improve the quality of your food, the quantity takes care of itself.

Every medical and nutrition expert I've ever trusted agrees that, for the most part, women do not need that much protein each day. I'm not saying that you should have carbohydrates at every meal, not by a long shot. I'm suggesting that you should have complex carbohydrates and vegetables for one meal and eat proteins (preferably fish or legumes and grains) with the proper vegetables at another. And if you *do* eat carbs and proteins together, eat a legume to link and balance the digestive process for the protein and starch. (A legume and a starch complement each other to make a complete protein.)

Why This Program Works as a Classic

It is so important to follow the basic guidelines of proper food combining. It is best to eat fruits by themselves, proteins and vegetables at one meal, and starches and vegetables at another meal. (See the charts on pages 94 and 95 for more detail and exceptions to the rules.) Food combining is not a diet. It's a way of life. And if you can do it as often as possible and follow the other Golden Rules of the Total Health Makeover, I promise you you will look and feel your best. I have never seen this *not* work. And that is why this way of eating is a classic. It is the best of many theories, combined with the conclusions I have reached from years of mistakes.

How These Recipes Were Chosen

The recipes in this book were chosen based on the following criteria:

1. No chemicals, especially no aspartame, nitrates, or nitrites.
2. No sugar. Sugar is really a chemical. None of these recipes contain refined white sugar. We use date sugar, maple syrup, maple sugar, honey, barley malt, rice syrup, fruit juice sweetener, and Sucanat and Rapadura, which are both made from sugar cane, but 98 percent of the nutrients have not been taken out, as they have been with white sugar. These are the only sweeteners that are used in the desserts or in some of the other recipes.

MARILU HENNER'S FOOD-COMBINING CHART

CHART 1

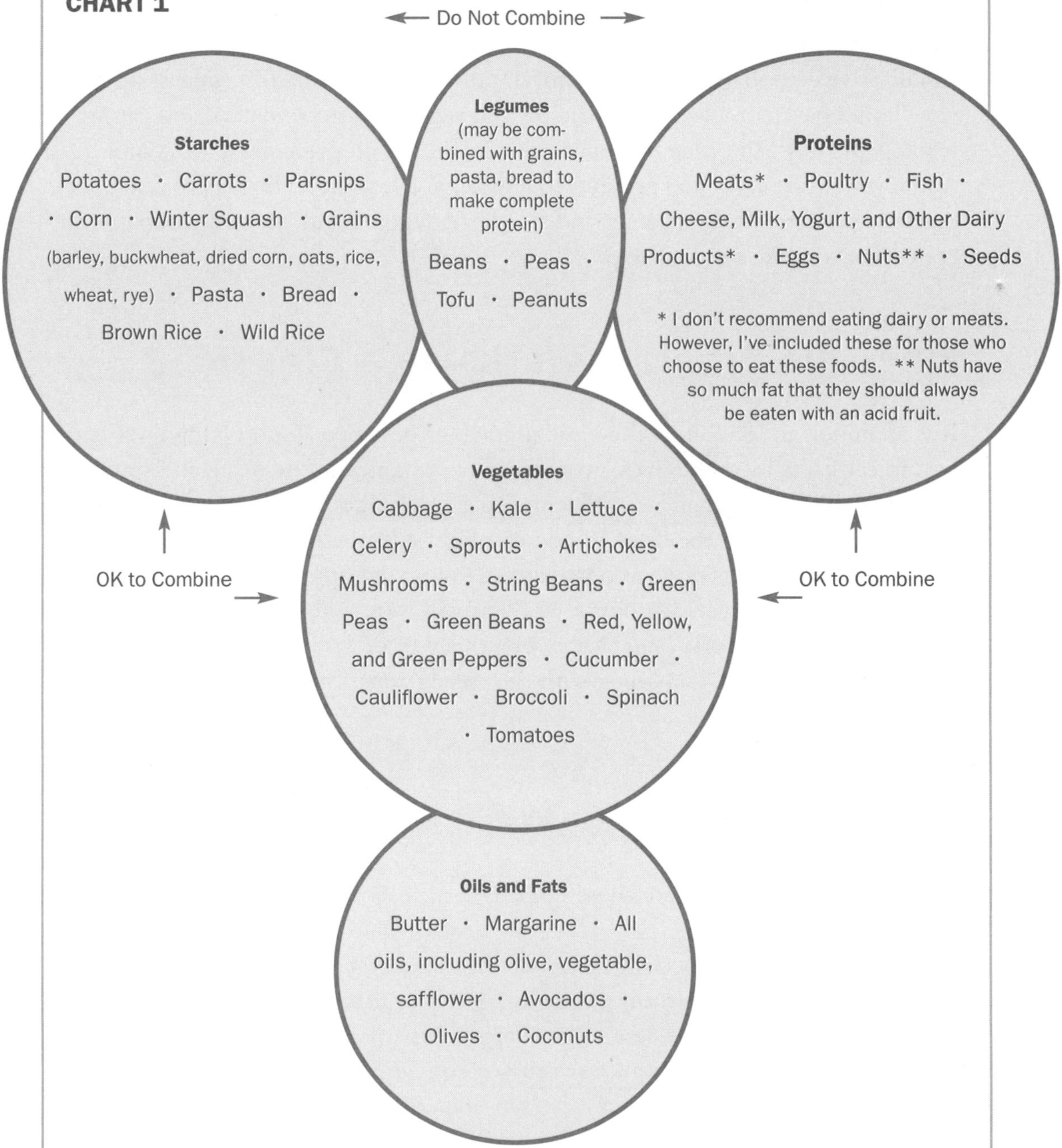

← Do Not Combine →

Starches

Potatoes · Carrots · Parsnips · Corn · Winter Squash · Grains (barley, buckwheat, dried corn, oats, rice, wheat, rye) · Pasta · Bread · Brown Rice · Wild Rice

Legumes

(may be combined with grains, pasta, bread to make complete protein)

Beans · Peas · Tofu · Peanuts

Proteins

Meats* · Poultry · Fish · Cheese, Milk, Yogurt, and Other Dairy Products* · Eggs · Nuts** · Seeds

* I don't recommend eating dairy or meats. However, I've included these for those who choose to eat these foods. ** Nuts have so much fat that they should always be eaten with an acid fruit.

OK to Combine →

OK to Combine ←

Vegetables

Cabbage · Kale · Lettuce · Celery · Sprouts · Artichokes · Mushrooms · String Beans · Green Peas · Green Beans · Red, Yellow, and Green Peppers · Cucumber · Cauliflower · Broccoli · Spinach · Tomatoes

Oils and Fats

Butter · Margarine · All oils, including olive, vegetable, safflower · Avocados · Olives · Coconuts

DO NOT COMBINE FOODS FROM CHART 1 AND 2

CHART 2

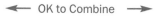 ← OK to Combine →

Acid Fruits

Grapefruits · Oranges ·
Lemons · Limes · Strawberries ·
Cranberries · Kiwis · Pineapples

Sub-Acid Fruits

Apples · Apricots · Blackberries
· Cherries · Peaches · Plums ·
Pears · Raspberries · Mangoes ·
Nectarines · Grapes · Papayas

Sweet Fruits

Bananas · Plantains ·
Dates · Persimmons · Figs
· Prunes · Raisins ·
Dried Fruits

Do not combine with
other foods

Melons

Cantaloupe · Honeydew ·
Watermelon · Casaba ·
Christmas · Crenshaw

Do not combine with other
foods

3. No dairy. There are no dairy products (including milk, cream, butter, cheese, yogurt, or whey) in *any* of these recipes. We use instead rice milk, soy milk, and margarine made with soybean oil.

4. No heavy meats. There's no red meat, pork, or veal in any of these dishes. Most of the protein dishes are made with fish, beans, legumes, tofu, and a limited amount of poultry (for those of you who eat chicken or turkey).

5. Fresh whole foods. We use foods that are natural and organic whenever possible, and, for the most part, these recipes follow the basic guidelines of proper food combining. See the food-combining charts on pages 94 and 95. They may not all follow the absolute rules of food combining, but the few dishes that veer off the track can be fixed with a legume dish.

The recipes were compiled from several sources. They are basically some of the best-loved recipes of the last twenty years from family, friends, and my all-time favorite restaurants, as well as the most outstanding dishes that were submitted to my website by people who have been on the program. My staff and I have been testing each and every one of these recipes over the last few months to make sure the balance and flavors (and instructions) of each dish are just right. You can just imagine how wonderful my kitchen has smelled. (My boys are going to expect this kind of culinary excitement from now on.) It's been a lot of fun for all of us as we've been cooking, tasting, and rating.

Key to Ratings and Symbols

Each recipe has a code based on cost, degree of difficulty, and in what week the recipe fits into *The 30-Day Total Health Makeover* for those of you who would like to swap out a recipe.

At the end of the book, on page 332, we've compiled categorical listings so you can find the perfect recipe for any situation. We've also put together the top ten favorites from each taster so you can see if you have a similar palate to anyone on our team. I hope you enjoy these recipes with as much gusto as I've had putting them together for you.

B.E.S.T of Health!

—Marilu

Cost	$	Under $5 per serving
	$$	$5 to $10 per serving
	$$$	Over $10 per serving *(as in a fish entrée)*
Degree of Difficulty	♟	Beginner
	♟♟	Intermediate
	♟♟♟	Advanced
Week	Yellow	Purple, Blue, Green, or Yellow *(refers to The 30-Day Total Health Makeover guidelines)*

7

Recipes

Breakfast

Jessica's Breakfast Smoothies

Jessica Prescott

SERVES 1

Jessica: *I start just about every day with this fast, simple, and delicious smoothie that is also portable for those extra-rushed mornings. The frozen mango I find at Trader Joe's. Any frozen fruit can be substituted. Peaches are another favorite.*

Marilu: *This is a great morning starter. You can make it with your favorite fruit and juice of choice.*

Tasters' comments: *"Good fast breakfast." "Out the door." "The boys loved them." "Good power drink."*

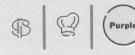

1 cup orange juice
5 cubes frozen mango
2 or 3 frozen strawberries

Put all ingredients into a blender and blend until smooth, about 45 to 60 seconds.

Blueberry Breakfast Frappe

Diane Beane

MAKES 1 SMOOTHIE

Diane: Here is my recipe for a wonderfully refreshing way to start your day!

Tasters' comments: "Delicious." "Light and easy to take on the go."
"Kids love them." "Lighter and easier to drink than Jamba Juice."
"Satisfying for your morning meal."

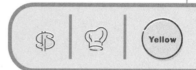

½ cup frozen blueberries

1 banana, sliced

½ cup soy or rice milk

1 ½ tablespoons raw honey

½ cup ice

Put ingredients together in a blender and mix until smooth. Garnish with a slice of banana.

Tip: Blueberries are a great antioxidant.

Coffee Cake Muffins

Marilu: These light, fluffy, sweet, delicious treats are not just for breakfast.

Tasters' comments: "Incredibly dangerous." "You want to eat the whole batch." "Kids will want them in their lunch boxes the next day."

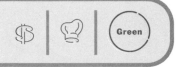

⅓ cup maple sugar

2 tablespoons soy margarine, softened

1 egg white, beaten

2⅓ cups organic unbleached flour

3½ teaspoons baking powder

2 teaspoons cinnamon

½ teaspoon sea salt

1 cup soy milk

1 teaspoon vanilla extract

Crunchy Topping

¼ cup soy margarine

½ cup maple sugar

⅓ cup organic unbleached flour

½ teaspoon cinnamon

In a mixing bowl, cream maple sugar and soy margarine. Add egg white; mix well. Combine flour, baking powder, cinnamon, and salt; add to the creamed mixture alternately with soy milk. Stir in vanilla. Fill 12 paper-lined muffin cups two-thirds full. In a small bowl, combine soy margarine, maple sugar, flour, and cinnamon until crumbly. Sprinkle evenly over muffins. Bake at 375 degrees for 25 to 30 minutes or until browned.

Cornmeal Flapjacks

SERVES 4

Marilu: These are so fluffy and light, we photographed them. They are fun to make with your kids. Best when made on an even heat source. Tastes just like what you'd get at your local breakfast spot.

Tasters' comments: "Great consistency." "Sweet enough to eat without syrup." "Good for freezing, just pop in the toaster to reheat."

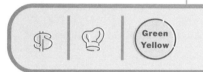

1 cup unbleached white flour
½ cup cornmeal
3 tablespoons Sucanat
2 teaspoons baking powder
1 teaspoon baking soda
½ cup soy milk

⅛ teaspoon salt
1¼ cups plain soy yogurt
2 large eggs
½ stick soy margarine, melted
Warm syrup

Whisk together flour, cornmeal, Sucanat, baking powder, baking soda, soy milk, and salt in a large bowl. Stir together soy yogurt and eggs with a fork in another bowl and stir into flour mixture with melted soy margarine just until incorporated.

Heat a lightly greased large nonstick skillet over moderately low heat until hot. Pour ¼ cup measures of batter into skillet in batches, forming 3 ½-inch cakes, and cook about 3 minutes, or until undersides are golden. Turn and cook 1 minute more, or until golden.

Transfer to a baking sheet and keep warm in a 250-degree oven while cooking remaining cakes.

Serve with warm syrup.

Sweet Potato Hash Browns

SERVES 4 TO 6

Marilu: The combination of sweet with regular potatoes is a great side with egg white dishes. It's a nice change from traditional hash browns.

Tasters' comments: "Good consistency." "Yum. Yum."

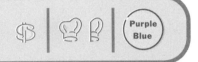

1 large sweet potato
2 large white potatoes
Oil spray

2 tablespoons olive oil
1 onion, sliced

Preheat oven to 400 degrees. Peel and chop potatoes. Spray a baking dish with oil to coat lightly. Lay potatoes in dish and bake for 15 minutes. In a skillet, heat olive oil, add onion, and cook until onion is golden brown. Add the potatoes from oven and stir. Serve hot.

Waffles, Pancakes, and Crepes

Denise Barker

Denise: I double this batch and freeze the waffles. My kids love them. They just pop them in the toaster.

Marilu: Breakfast at its best. This batter is so fluffy and delicious. It makes a wonderful lower-fat alternative if you use less oil.

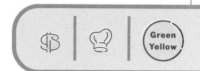

⅓ cup olive oil (I find this a bit strong so I decrease a bit and increase the apple juice and milk substitute)

¾ cup Rice Dream

¾ cup apple juice

2 eggs

2 cups flour of choice (rice flour works best because it gives a slightly crispier texture—I use half brown rice flour and half white rice flour)

1 teaspoon baking powder

Mix the wet ingredients together, then add the dry and mix well. To make crepes you will need the batter thinner, so add more apple juice. Heat your waffle iron or skillet and go!

Soy Cheese and Mushroom Frittata

SERVES 4 TO 6

Marilu: *This versatile frittata is a wonderful brunch dish. You can try your favorite veggies and substitute egg whites. Sliced on a plate it also looks very impressive.*

Tasters' comments: *"Old European taste at your table."*

Green
Yellow

2 tablespoons soy margarine
⅓ cup thinly sliced shallots (1 large)
Freshly ground black pepper to taste
2 cups fresh oyster mushrooms or
    other wild mushrooms, cut into
    ½-inch strips

8 eggs
2 tablespoons chopped fresh parsley
3 to 4 ounces soy cheddar or
    mozzarella, grated

Preheat the broiler.

Melt the margarine in a 10-inch flameproof skillet. Stir in the shallots and pepper. Cook over medium-high heat, stirring, until the shallots are golden, about 2 minutes. Then stir in the mushrooms, and cook 1 minute.

Lightly beat eggs, add parsley, and season with pepper. Add grated soy cheese. Lower the heat to medium-low and pour mixture into the skillet. Stir quickly, incorporating the mushroom mixture. Cook until the bottom is set; the top should still be wet, 3 to 4 minutes.

Place the skillet under the broiler and cook until the frittata is sizzling, puffed, and set, 1 to 2 minutes. Serve immediately.

Blueberry Crunch Muffins

Marisol Rippy

MAKES 12 MUFFINS

Marilu: *These sweet cakes taste so sinful, you can't believe they work within the program's rules. They're great to put in kids' lunches.*

Taster's comments: *"A melody in your mouth."*
"Unbelievably moist."

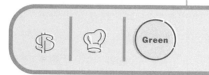

⅓ cup Sucanat

¼ cup soy margarine, softened

1 egg white, beaten

2 cups organic unbleached flour

3½ teaspoons baking powder

½ teaspoon sea salt

1 cup soy milk

1 teaspoon vanilla extract

1½ cups frozen or fresh organic blueberries

Crunchy Topping

¼ cup soy margarine

½ cup Sucanat

⅓ cup organic unbleached flour

½ teaspoon cinnamon

In a mixing bowl, cream Sucanat and soy margarine. Add egg white; mix well. In another bowl combine flour, baking powder, and salt; add to the creamed mixture alternately with soy milk. Stir in vanilla. Fold in blueberries. Fill 12 paper-lined muffin cups two-thirds full. In a small bowl, combine soy margarine, Sucanat, flour, and cinnamon until crumbly. Sprinkle evenly over muffins. Bake at 375 degrees for 25 to 30 minutes or until browned.

Maple Danish

Marilu: These are great for a Sunday brunch. You can experiment with other uses for the dough and add poppy seeds or maple for variety. They look very pretty on the table.

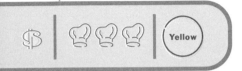

Dough
1 package active dry yeast
4 tablespoons Sucanat
1 cup warm water
2 cups unbleached white flour

After First Rise
½ cup oil
¼ cup Sucanat
1 teaspoon salt
1½ cups unbleached white flour

Tofu Filling
½ cup water
2 tablespoons oil
⅓ cup soy milk
1 cup crumbled soft tofu
¼ cup fresh lemon juice
½ cup maple sugar
½ teaspoon salt

2 tablespoons unbleached white flour
Oil for brushing the dough

Start the dough: Dissolve the yeast and 1 tablespoon of the Sucanat in the warm water. Let stand 5 minutes, then mix in the flour and the remaining 3 tablespoons Sucanat. Beat well and let rise until doubled, about an hour.

Dissolve together the oil, ¼ cup Sucanat, and the salt. Mix this into the flour and yeast mixture with your hands. Add 1½ cups flour to make a kneadable dough.

Knead until smooth and soft, but not sticky. Let rise for an hour, or until dough has doubled.

To make the filling, in a blender combine the water, oil, soy milk, and tofu until smooth and creamy. Pour this into a small saucepan and whisk in the lemon juice, maple sugar, and salt. Cook over medium heat, stirring constantly, until thickened. Remove from heat and cool before filling the danish dough.

Preheat oven to 350 degrees. Sprinkle a little flour on your work surface and roll the dough about ⅛ inch thick. Brush with oil and cut into 4 x 4-inch squares. Place 1 scant tablespoon of filling in the center of each square. Fold two opposite corners of the dough toward the middle and pinch together. Take the remaining unfolded corners and curl them in toward the filling. Let rise 5 minutes. Place on a well-oiled cookie sheet. Leave ½ to 1 inch space between each danish. Bake for about 15 minutes or until light golden brown. Brush with oil for last 3 minutes of baking.

Polenta French Toast

Bread & Butter Catering

SERVES 6

Marilu: Bread & Butter is one of my favorite caterers. Chef Michael Brooks is never afraid to experiment and always comes through. This fancy version of French toast is truly impressive at a brunch. The best thing is that you can make it the night before and slice the following morning.

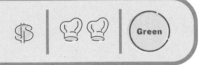

2 quarts vanilla soy milk

2 tablespoons soy margarine plus
    more for sautéing

2 cups coarse stone-ground yellow
    cornmeal

4 tablespoons maple syrup

½ cup golden raisins

Bring soy milk and soy margarine to a boil in heavy medium saucepan, slowly whisk in cornmeal and stir constantly for 8 to 10 minutes until mixture is thickened and starts to pull away from the sides. Add maple syrup, stir until combined, then add raisins. Pour into an 8½ x 4½-inch loaf pan. Fill to the top and discard any excess. Smooth top with a spatula and place in refrigerator until chilled.

Invert pan onto cutting board and slice polenta into 12 wedges.

Heat a griddle or a cast-iron pan. Add soy margarine and sauté wedges until golden brown on both sides.

Banana Bread

MAKES 1 LOAF

Marilu: This bread has versatility, depending on the flour you use. With wheat flour, it's more of a bread than a "sweet" bread, and very hearty. If you make it with regular flour, make extra for muffins; kids love it in their lunch.

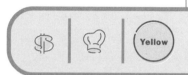

8 tablespoons soy margarine, room temperature
¾ cup Sucanat
2 eggs
1 cup unbleached all-purpose flour
1 teaspoon baking soda

½ teaspoon salt
1 cup whole wheat flour or unbleached all-purpose flour
3 large, ripe bananas, mashed
1 teaspoon vanilla extract

Preheat oven to 350 degrees. Grease a 9 x 5 x 3-inch bread pan.

Cream soy margarine and Sucanat until light and fluffy. Add eggs, one at a time, beating well after each addition.

Sift all-purpose flour, baking soda, and salt together, stir in whole wheat flour and add to creamed mixture, mixing well. Fold in bananas and vanilla.

Pour mixture into the prepared pan. Bake for 50 to 60 minutes, or until a cake tester inserted in the center comes out clean. Cool in pan for 10 minutes, then on rack.

Zucchini Bread

Marilu: *This recipe was made more than any other during the course of working on this book. I like to use date sugar instead of Sucanat. For best flavor, wrap the bread when cool and let stand overnight before serving. With its spices and nuts, this is a tea bread, almost cakelike.*

Tasters' comments: *"It's fantastic." "It cooks perfectly."*

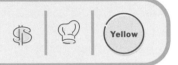

3 eggs

1 cup oil

1½ cups Sucanat

1 teaspoon vanilla extract

2 cups grated, unpeeled raw zucchini

2 cups unbleached all-purpose flour

2 teaspoons baking soda

2 teaspoons baking powder

1 teaspoon salt

½ teaspoon ground cinnamon

½ teaspoon ground cloves

Preheat oven to 350 degrees. Butter a 9 x 5-inch loaf pan.

Beat eggs, oil, Sucanat, and vanilla until light and thick. Fold grated zucchini into oil mixture.

Sift dry ingredients together. Stir into zucchini mixture until just blended. Pour into the buttered loaf pan. Bake on middle rack of oven for 1 hour and 15 minutes, or until a cake tester inserted in the center comes out clean.

Cool slightly, remove from pan, and cool completely on a rack.

Appetizers

Wild Mushroom Bruschetta

Marilu: This dish reminded most of us of our favorite Italian restaurants. It has a rustic, Tuscan flavor. Great the next day too.

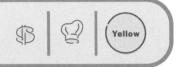

Twelve 3 x 2 x ¼-inch diagonal slices French-bread baguette
3 tablespoons olive oil
Salt and pepper
3 tablespoons soy margarine
1½ pounds fresh wild mushrooms (such as crimini, oyster, and stemmed shiitake), chopped

⅓ cup finely chopped shallots
5 minced garlic cloves
2 tablespoons chopped fresh parsley
1 teaspoon chopped fresh thyme, or ½ teaspoon dried
1 teaspoon chopped fresh marjoram, or ½ teaspoon dried
3 cups dry white wine

Preheat oven to 350 degrees. Place bread slices on baking sheet. Brush with 1 tablespoon olive oil and sprinkle with salt and pepper. Bake until bread just begins to color, about 8 minutes. Remove from oven and let cool.

Melt 2 tablespoons soy margarine with remaining 2 tablespoons olive oil in heavy large skillet over medium-high heat until soy margarine is golden brown, about 2 minutes. Add mushrooms and sauté until golden, about 8 minutes. Add shallots, garlic, and herbs and sauté 2 minutes. Add wine and simmer until mushrooms are tender and juices thicken enough to coat mushrooms, about 25 minutes. Add remaining 1 tablespoon soy margarine; stir until margarine melts. Divide wild mushroom mixture equally among 12 toasts.

Tip: When you finely chop the mushrooms, it brings out more flavor.

Classic Bruschetta

Marilu: This is one of those crowd-pleasing appetizers. It's easy to make and great when guests want to join you in the kitchen.

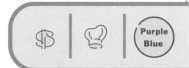

8 plum tomatoes, chopped and
   seeded

8 basil leaves, chopped

1 to 2 garlic cloves, minced

2 teaspoons olive oil

Salt and pepper to taste

1 French baguette, sliced thin and
   toasted

Mix all ingredients except the bread. Spoon on top of bread and serve.

Stuffed Mushrooms

Marilu: Fantastic. This dish fooled our most polluted friends. A great appetizer that's easy to eat standing. Try to walk away. You'll be back.

Tasters' comments: "It tastes like it's bad for you."

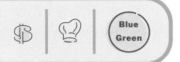

12 fresh white button mushrooms at least 2 inches in diameter

2 tablespoons extra-virgin olive oil, plus extra for drizzling

2 green scallions

2 large cloves garlic, finely chopped or passed through a garlic press

2½ tablespoons chopped fresh Italian parsley

¼ cup fine dried bread crumbs

3 tablespoons soy Parmesan

½ teaspoon minced fresh oregano, or ¼ teaspoon dried oregano

¼ teaspoon salt

Freshly ground black pepper

1 tablespoon dry vermouth (optional)

Preheat oven to 375 degrees. Using a soft brush or clean kitchen towel, remove any dirt from the mushrooms. Do not wash them because water alters their texture. Trim off the rough bottom from each stem and discard; only the rest of the stem will be used. Separate the stems at the base of the caps of 9 of the mushrooms. Chop all of the stems along with the 3 remaining whole mushrooms.

In a skillet over medium heat, warm the 2 tablespoons olive oil. Add the scallions, garlic, and parsley and sauté gently until wilted, about 4 minutes. Add the chopped mushrooms and sauté gently until softened, about 5 minutes more. Remove the mixture to a small bowl. Add the bread crumbs, soy Parmesan, oregano, salt, and pepper to taste to the mushroom mixture and mix well.

Fill each mushroom cap with an equal amount of the stuffing, using your hands to form the stuffing into a nice even mound and to push it down to fill the underside of the caps. Place the filled mushrooms on a baking sheet. Sprinkle the vermouth over the mushrooms if using, and then drizzle each mushroom very lightly with olive oil.

Cover loosely with aluminum foil and bake for 20 minutes. Remove the foil and bake until the mushrooms are bubbling and golden, an additional 10 to 15 minutes. Serve hot or warm.

Note: The mushrooms can be stuffed up to a day in advance, then covered and refrigerated until ready to bake. Sprinkle with the vermouth and olive oil just before baking.

Olive's Tuna Tartare

Todd English

Marilu: While performing in Vegas last summer, I fell in love with Olive's Restaurant at the Bellagio Hotel. Here's my favorite dish. I've been known to order two of these in one sitting—one for an appetizer and one for dinner. Yes, it's that good.

Blue Green

1½ pounds very fresh bluefin or yellowfin tuna, diced into pieces the size of a raisin

1 tablespoon chopped fresh basil leaves

1 tablespoon chopped fresh cilantro leaves

1 tablespoon finely chopped peeled fresh ginger

Greens from 1 bunch scallions, finely chopped

½ to 1 teaspoon Vietnamese chili paste

2 teaspoons soy sauce

½ teaspoon black pepper

1 to 2 teaspoons kosher salt

2 tablespoons extra-virgin olive oil

1 teaspoon roasted sesame oil

Combine all the ingredients in a large bowl. Cover and chill for no longer than 1 hour before serving.

Serve on fresh sliced cucumbers if food-combining, or on toast points if including a bean dish with your meal.

Note: If you cannot find Vietnamese chili paste, you can substitute Chinese or Thai chili paste, which you should be able to find in any well-stocked grocery store. Because different brands vary in degrees of hotness, you should add a small amount at a time and taste after each addition.

Border Grill's Ceviche de Veracruz

Susan Feniger

SERVES 4 TO 6

Susan: Flavorful, meaty bits of swordfish or mussels go well with this strong marinade from coastal Veracruz.

Marilu: I like this dish served like a seafood martini. Make extra, it tastes great the next day.

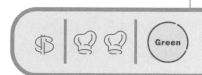

10 ounces fresh swordfish, cut into ½-inch cubes, or shelled mussels

½ cup plus 1 tablespoon freshly squeezed lime juice

1 small red onion, diced

2 medium tomatoes, cored, seeded, and diced

½ cup freshly squeezed orange juice

½ cup tomato juice

2 jalapeño chiles, stemmed, seeded, and finely chopped

1 bunch fresh oregano, leaves only, chopped (about ½ cup)

¼ cup extra-virgin olive oil

½ cup small green olives, pitted

1 teaspoon salt

½ teaspoon pepper

Lettuce leaves for serving

Combine the fish or mussels and ½ cup of the lime juice in a glass or ceramic dish and marinate for 30 minutes in the refrigerator. Drain and discard the lime juice.

Transfer the fish to a medium bowl. Add the remaining 1 tablespoon of lime juice, the onion, tomatoes, orange juice, tomato juice, chiles, oregano, olive oil, olives, salt, and pepper. Toss well and chill for at least an hour, or as long as overnight. Serve cold in chilled glasses or on lettuce-lined plates.

Warning: Be careful not to overmarinate the fish in the initial lime juice. If the fish is left in too long, lime can overcook the fish's fibers, turning them to mush.

Summer Wrap

Marilu: This wrap would impress Martha Stewart. It looks beautiful and healthy. The taste and texture balance is something else. Make extra—it's great for lunch.

Tasters' comments: "Fresh and delicious with snap."

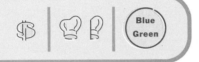

20 asparagus stalks

1 avocado

Juice of ½ lime

Salt and pepper to taste

2 cups cooked brown rice

2 tablespoons soy yogurt

3 tablespoons Nayonaise

¼ teaspoon chili oil

Pinch of chili powder

Pinch of sweet cayenne

5 whole wheat tortillas

½ cup cilantro

½ cup chopped red onion

Steam asparagus in a steamer basket within a medium pot with 2 inches of water for 5 to 7 minutes, so asparagus stays firm. Remove from heat, set aside.

In a separate bowl, mash avocado and lime juice. Add salt and pepper to taste.

In another bowl, mix brown rice and soy yogurt. In yet another bowl, mix Nayonaise, chili oil, chili powder, and cayenne (adjust spice according to taste).

On a clean, dry surface, lay out tortillas. Spread pepper and Nayonaise mixture thinly over surface of tortillas, then avocado mixture, brown rice, cilantro and onion, and finally asparagus. Fold tortillas, wrap in plastic wrap, and chill for 25 minutes.

After chilling, remove plastic wrap and cut each wrap twice, diagonally (to make three pieces). Serve cold.

Shrimp and Black Bean Lettuce Wrap

Bryony and Inara SERVES 4 TO 6

Marilu: This Asian-influenced Tex-Mex flavor actually happened by accident during one of those "I'm in the mood for this flavor" kind of moments.

Tasters' comments: "Wonderful combo of the sweetness in scallions and cilantro." "Fun to eat."

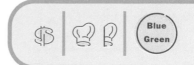

2 tablespoons olive oil

1 teaspoon chili pepper

1 teaspoon ginger, fresh or dried

1 pound fresh rock shrimp, shelled
   and cleaned

1 cup chopped red onions

Salt and pepper to taste

One 10-ounce can black beans

1 cup chopped scallions

1 cup chopped cilantro

1 head butter lettuce, cleaned and
   separated

Heat 1 tablespoon of olive oil with chili pepper and ginger over low heat. Add shrimp to mixture and turn heat to medium-low. Sauté until shrimp turn pink, about 8 minutes. Set aside. In a separate skillet, sauté red onions in 1 tablespoon olive oil over medium-low heat for 5 minutes. Add salt and pepper to taste. Add one-third of the black beans, sauté, and mash the beans. Add remaining beans, sauté, leaving those beans whole.

Add shrimp mixture, scallions, and cilantro. Sauté for 2 additional minutes.

Serve wrapped in butter lettuce or in a bowl so each individual can wrap his or her own.

Stuffed Zucchini

Marilu: *This is a great dish when you're in the mood for something "cheesy." It tastes like it's bad for you.*

Tasters' comments: *"Fantastic."*

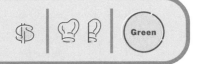

4 young, tender zucchini (6 to
  8 ounces each)
Salt
¼ pound stale bread, crusts removed
⅓ cup soy milk
¼ pound fresh white button
  mushrooms
3 tablespoons olive oil
2 large cloves garlic, finely
  chopped or passed through a garlic
  press

1 small onion, chopped
3 tablespoons chopped fresh Italian
  parsley
2 teaspoons chopped fresh
  marjoram, or 1 teaspoon dried
  marjoram
1 egg, lightly beaten
Freshly ground black pepper
7 tablespoons soy Parmesan

Preheat oven to 400 degrees.

Wash the zucchini well to remove any embedded dirt. Fill a large saucepan with water and bring to a boil. Add 1 tablespoon salt and the zucchini and boil until they are just tender but not too soft, about 10 minutes.

Meanwhile, shred the bread and place it in a small bowl with the soy milk to soak. Using a soft brush or clean kitchen towel, remove any dirt from the mushrooms. Trim off the bottoms from the stems and discard. Quarter the mushrooms and slice them thinly.

As soon as the zucchini are ready, drain them. When cool enough to handle, trim off their ends. Cut them in half lengthwise. With a paring knife, scoop out the flesh, leaving a shell about ¼ inch thick. Using your hands, wring out as much water as possible from the scooped out flesh. Chop it up and set it aside.

Place the oil, garlic, and onion in a cold skillet over low heat. Sauté gently until the garlic and onion are softened but not colored, about 7 minutes. Add the parsley and sauté for an additional minute. Add the sliced mushrooms and marjoram to the skillet and sauté gently until the mushrooms are softened, about 8 minutes. Transfer to a bowl.

When the mushroom mixture has cooled, add the egg, ¾ teaspoon salt, pepper to taste, and 6 tablespoons of the soy Parmesan. Using your hands, squeeze out as much of the soy milk as possible from the bread. Add it and the chopped zucchini flesh to the mushroom mixture and mix thoroughly. Spoon the mixture into the zucchini shells, dividing it equally among them. Place the stuffed zucchini in a baking dish and sprinkle the remaining 1 tablespoon soy Parmesan over them.

Slip the dish onto the middle rack of the oven and bake until golden, about 30 minutes. Serve hot, warm, or at room temperature.

Coconut Shrimp with Curried Hummus on Wonton Squares

Bread & Butter Catering

MAKES 30 TO 40 SQUARES

Marilu: This is one of my favorite appetizers ever. And believe it or not, it works within the food-combining rules because of the beans. Enjoy this beautiful blend of flavors and textures!

1 package wonton wrappers

Canola oil for frying

½ cup tahini

½ cup olive oil

Curried Hummus

One 16-ounce can garbanzo beans, rinsed and drained

¼ cup warm water

2 tablespoons curry powder

2 teaspoons turmeric

Coconut Shrimp

1 cup honey

2 cups sweetened coconut

1 pound medium raw shrimp (30 to 40 count), tails off, cleaned and cut in half

Cut wonton wrappers into quarters. Pour 2 inches of canola oil into frying pan and heat until hot but not smoking. Fry wonton squares 6 or so at a time, turning once, until golden brown. Drain on paper towels.

To make hummus, place garbanzo beans in a food processor and with machine running, add warm water. Add other ingredients with machine running until well blended and smooth.

Preheat oven to 350 degrees.

Place honey and coconut in two separate bowls. Dip shrimp halves first in honey, then coconut, then place on foil-covered baking sheet. Bake shrimp until just pink and cooked through.

Meanwhile, spread a small amount of hummus on each wonton square. Using tongs, place hot shrimp on wontons. Serve immediately.

Wild Rice Pancakes

Bread & Butter Catering   MAKES 15 TO 20 THREE-INCH PANCAKES

Marilu: *An interesting and flavorful twist on potato pancakes. A real crowd pleaser. Serve at a party and watch them disappear.*

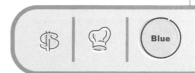

1 cup flour

2 tablespoons baking powder

2 tablespoons dried onions

1½ cups soy milk

Vegetarian egg substitute to equal
   3 eggs

2 dashes Tabasco sauce

2 dashes Worcestershire sauce

⅔ cup cooked wild rice

Soy margarine to coat the griddle

Sift together flour, baking powder, and onions. Whisk in soy milk, egg substitute, Tabasco, and Worcestershire. Fold in wild rice.

Heat griddle or cast-iron skillet to medium-high, melt soy margarine, and spoon batter onto hot surface. Cook until browned, flip, and cook until browned on the other side.

Notes: Serve with organic applesauce for a savory breakfast.

Add a little black pepper and 1 chopped Red Delicious apple for a wonderful topping on appetizer-size pancakes.

If you want to serve this as an entrée, make 6 to 8 large pancakes.

Chilled Tofu with Scallion-Citrus Marinade

Spencer Gray

SERVES 4

Marilu: This Asian-inspired dish is for the "purist." You can taste all of the flavors. It's light and healthy and it looks pretty. It even has a little kick.

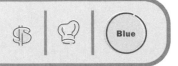

6 scallions

1 bunch cilantro, finely minced

1 bunch parsley, finely minced

Juice of 1 lime

3 tablespoons extra-virgin olive oil

2 tablespoons sesame oil

2 tablespoons rice wine vinegar

2 tablespoons soy sauce

Salt and pepper

One 1-pound block extra-firm tofu, not the silken kind because it falls apart

Garnish: chili-garlic paste and fried leeks

Trim ⅔ of white part from scallions and reserve for another use. Finely mince remainder of white ends and green portions of scallions. Add equal amount of cilantro, and about one-third that amount of parsley. Put in mixing bowl.

Add to the mixture the lime juice, olive oil, sesame oil, rice wine vinegar, and 1 tablespoon soy sauce. Mix well until herbs are fully coated and mixture resembles a paste. Let sit at room temperature for about ½ hour. Add salt and pepper to suit your palate.

Slice tofu in half crosswise. Placing each piece on its side, cut again in half until you have four flat, even slabs. On a small plate, spread a thin layer of chili-garlic paste a little larger than the dimensions of your tofu slab. Place tofu slab over chili-garlic paste. Spread a thin layer of the herb marinade evenly over tofu, and cut tofu into even 1-inch blocks. Sprinkle with leeks julienned into 2-inch strips and flash-fried. Serve.

Notes: This dish is a study in contrasts between the cool mildness of the tofu and the light crispness of the leeks, between the spice of the chili-garlic paste and the fresh acidity of the marinade, the bright green of the herbs and the scarlet fire of the chili paste. Your end result should be light, refreshing, spicy, and cool.

Since everything is raw, the quality of your ingredients is crucial. Look for the freshest, greenest herbs. I recommend curly parsley over the Italian flat-leafed variety because it is milder and will not overwhelm the cilantro. Also a fruity, clean olive oil with fresh olive flavor and a good green hue will add depth and brightness to your dish. In the same vein, be sure to use a sesame oil that is full, nutty, and not diluted with lesser oils.

Stuffed Grape Leaves with Lemon Sauce

Denise Barker

SERVES 6

Denise: I'm taking this to my New Year's Eve party.

Marilu: Next time you have to bring a dish to a friend's house, bring this and they'll be impressed.

Tasters' comments: "The lemon sauce makes the grape leaves dance."

Green Yellow

Rice Pilaf

1½ cups raw brown rice, short or long grain

2¼ cups water

2 tablespoons olive oil

1½ cups finely chopped onion

1 small celery stalk, chopped fine

½ teaspoon salt

½ cup toasted pine nuts or sunflower seeds

Black pepper to taste

4 to 5 medium cloves garlic, finely chopped

2 tablespoons lemon juice

¼ cup fresh chopped parsley

1 tablespoon dried mint, or 3 tablespoons fresh chopped mint

24 grape leaves, 3 to 4 inches across (I rinse mine, as they are very salty when they come out of the jar)

Lemon Sauce

1 box firm silken tofu (10½ ounces)

1 tablespoon fresh lemon juice

½ teaspoon salt

A few dashes of pepper

Place rice and water in a saucepan and bring to a boil. Cover and reduce heat so the water and rice simmer gently. Cook for approximately 40 minutes or until cooked. In a large frying pan, heat the olive oil and sauté the onion, celery, and salt until the vegetables are tender.

Now add the toasted nuts or seeds, pepper, and garlic. Sauté for an additional

5 minutes. Once the rice is cooked, add the sautéed vegetables to it along with the lemon juice, parsley, and mint. Stir well. This can be used as a filling for grape leaves, artichokes, or eggplant. It is also delicious served on its own.

To prepare the grape leaves, lightly oil a baking tray. Place each leaf down flat on a clean surface. Place a heaping tablespoon of pilaf near the stem end of the leaf, then roll tightly, folding the sides in. Arrange the stuffed leaves on the baking tray. Bake at 325 degrees for about 20 minutes, or until heated through.

For the lemon sauce, blend all ingredients in a food processor or blender until smooth. Store in a tightly covered container in the refrigerator.

Note: This can be served as a main dish or appetizer. The stuffed grape leaves can be served cold as well, with the sauce on the side. If you have access to fresh grape leaves, they should be picked early in the season to insure their tenderness. Make sure they are large enough to stuff. Most people buy the grape leaves in a specialty food shop (my regular grocery store carries them in the imported food section).

Grilled Polenta Triangles with Sun-Dried Tomato Pesto and Oregano

Bread & Butter Catering   SERVES 30

Marilu: Lots of flavor and beautiful to look at. A feisty, festive, fabulous dish.

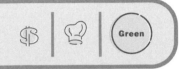

Polenta

2 quarts soy milk

2 tablespoons soy margarine

2 cups coarse stone-ground yellow cornmeal

1½ cups soy Parmesan

Sun-Dried Tomato Pesto

One 28-ounce can tomato puree

3 tablespoons extra-virgin olive oil

2 cloves garlic, minced

1½ cups sun-dried tomatoes, packed in oil, coarsely chopped

Soy margarine for frying

Fresh oregano leaves for garnish

Bring soy milk and soy margarine to a boil in heavy medium saucepan, slowly whisk in cornmeal, and stir constantly for 8 to 10 minutes until mixture is thickened and starts to pull away from the sides. Add soy Parmesan and stir until combined.

Put in the refrigerator to cool.

Invert onto cutting board, cut into 12 wedges, then cut each wedge into 8 triangles.

To make the pesto, place tomato puree, olive oil, and garlic in a sauté pan and cook over medium heat until thickened and slightly reduced (about 45 minutes), stirring occasionally.

Remove from heat. Stir in sun-dried tomatoes. Puree in a blender or food processor until smooth (makes 2½ cups).

Heat soy margarine on a griddle or in a cast-iron skillet until hot, but not smoking, and fry polenta until crispy and golden on both sides.

Top with a small dollop of pesto and garnish with 1 leaf fresh oregano.

Fondue 2000

Elizabeth Carney

SERVES 4 TO 6

Marilu: Elizabeth Carney is my talented and beautiful niece who not only writes and produces, but cooks like a chef. Here is something she came up with especially for this book. This soy cheese fondue is strongly similar to regular cheese fondue. Very festive, and it pleased one of our polluted panelists' palates. Just think, you can have a swinging seventies party all over again.

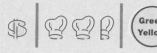

12 ounces Soya Kaas (it melts the best) Monterey Jack cheese

3 to 4 ounces Soya Kaas mild cheddar cheese

4 ounces soy Parmesan

1 tablespoon olive oil

½ cup vermouth

Bread cubes for serving

Apple slices for serving

Cut cheeses into ½-inch cubes. In double boiler or fondue pot, combine Parmesean, olive oil, and cheese cubes, adding the cubes slowly while stirring constantly. Add a little vermouth to keep it in a liquid consistency. Serve immediately with bread or apples. Keep it hot as long as you are eating. Once it's cold, it's like chocolate—it can't be reheated.

Tricolored Vegetable Pâté

SERVES 8

Marilu: This beautiful, sure-fire winner is a favorite with all of my friends. It gets requested every year. Make sure you save room for other food.

   Green Yellow

Squash Layer

1 butternut squash (about 1½ to 2 pounds)

2 tablespoons soy margarine

¼ cup Rice Dream

2 tablespoons flour

¼ teaspoon ground cinnamon

¼ teaspoon ground ginger

½ teaspoon salt

3 egg whites (or 2 eggs), lightly beaten

Mushroom Layer

¼ cup soy margarine

1 pound mushrooms, finely chopped (4 cups)

1 large onion, finely chopped (1 cup)

1 teaspoon salt

¼ teaspoon freshly ground black pepper

3 egg whites (or 2 eggs), lightly beaten

¼ cup packaged bread crumbs

Broccoli Layer

2 packages (10 ounces each) frozen chopped broccoli

2 tablespoons soy margarine

1 medium-size onion, finely chopped (½ cup)

1 clove garlic, finely chopped

½ cup Rice Dream

4 egg whites (or 3 eggs)

⅛ teaspoon ground nutmeg

¼ cup packaged bread crumbs

½ teaspoon salt

Watercress for garnish

Peel and cut squash into cubes and place in a large saucepan. Cover with boiling salted water and return to boil. Cover and simmer until very tender, about 30 minutes. Drain and puree in an electric blender or food processor.

In a medium saucepan, melt the soy margarine, stir in pureed squash, Rice Dream, flour, cinnamon, ginger, and salt. Cook, stirring, until mixture thickens and bubbles. Remove from heat and stir in the egg whites or eggs. Turn into a greased 9 x 5 x 3-inch loaf pan lined on the bottom and sides with foil.

Heat the soy margarine and sauté the mushrooms and onion until tender and most of the moisture has evaporated. Off the heat, stir in salt, pepper, egg whites or eggs, and bread crumbs. Place on top of squash mixture.

Cook the broccoli according to package directions. Drain and chop finely. Place in a bowl.

Meanwhile, heat the soy margarine in a small saucepan and saute the onion until tender but not browned. Add garlic and cook 1 minute. Add to broccoli.

Preheat oven to 350 degrees. Add Rice Dream, egg whites or eggs, nutmeg, bread crumbs, and salt to broccoli. Mix well and place on top of mushroom mixture. Place loaf pan in a 13 x 9 x 2-inch baking pan in the middle of the oven. Pour boiling water into outer pan to a depth of about 2 inches. Bake at 350 degrees for 2 hours or until pâté is set. Remove loaf pan to a wire rack to cool. Chill several hours or overnight.

Unmold onto a platter and garnish with watercress, if you wish.

Grilled Portobello Mushrooms with Sautéed Oyster Mushrooms

a tavola

SERVES 6

a tavola: This mushroom recipe has been on a tavola's menu from the first and has remained to this day because of its simply delicious appeal to vegetarians and nonvegetarians alike.

Tasters' comments: "Mushrooms are my favorite flavor."

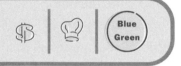

Oyster mushrooms	Portobello mushrooms
3 tablespoons extra-virgin olive oil	**6 cloves garlic, peeled**
1 pound oyster mushrooms	**3 sprigs rosemary**
6 sprigs fresh thyme	**12 leaves sage**
2 splashes white wine	**Small handful fresh thyme sprigs**
⅛ teaspoon kosher salt	**½ cup balsamic vinegar**
Freshly ground black pepper to taste	**Salt and pepper to taste**
	1½ cups extra-virgin olive oil
	6 portobello mushrooms, stemmed

Oyster mushrooms: In a very hot 10-inch frying pan, add olive oil and oyster mushrooms and toss. Add thyme and white wine and cook rapidly for approximately 1 minute. Add salt and cook for another minute. Taste the mushrooms for seasoning. The mushrooms are done when the raw taste is cooked out.

Portobello mushrooms: Roughly chop the garlic and herbs. Place in a large bowl and add the vinegar. Season the vinegar with salt and pepper, then whisk in the oil to make a vinaigrette. Lay the portobellos in a shallow baking dish and pour the vinaigrette over them. Cover and refrigerate overnight. Before serving, grill the portobellos over an open fire for approximately 3 minutes on each side or until the centers of the mushrooms are soft.

Arrange oyster mushrooms on a serving platter. Slice the portobellos at an angle and lay on the platter with the oyster mushrooms.

Smooth and Chunky Salsa

Bryony and Inara

MAKES 4 CUPS

Marilu: This has a traditional Mexican "smoky" flavor like cooked salsa. You can taste the spices, not just the "hot." It's so easy to whip up, and if you cook a lot, you most likely have all the ingredients you need. Maybe even the chips.

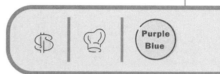

4 cups chopped tomatoes (plum, yellow, or any fresh variety)

1½ cups chopped cilantro

1 small Bermuda onion, chopped

Juice of ½ lime

Salt and pepper to taste

After all the vegetables are chopped, combine tomatoes, cilantro, and onion in a large bowl. Put half of everything into a food processor or blender with the lime juice. When it's finely pureed, pour back into original mixture and combine well. Add salt and pepper generously and refrigerate for ½ hour so the flavors mesh. Add more salt and pepper according to desired taste.

Guacamole

Bryony and Inara

Marilu: This smooth-textured guacamole is fresher tasting than store-bought or restaurant. There is something so satisfying about making your own.

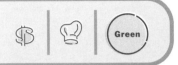

4 large Haas avocados, peeled and
    pitted
3 plum tomatoes, chopped
½ small Bermuda onion

½ cup chopped cilantro
1½ tablespoons lemon juice
Salt and pepper to taste

Combine all ingredients in a large bowl and mix/smash together. Salt and pepper generously.

Spicy Guacamole

Bryony and Inara

MAKES 2 CUPS

Marilu: *Nothing is better than guacamole with a little kick to it. I love spicy anything, and this really hits the spot.*

Tasters' comments: *"I wanted to eat the whole bowl."*

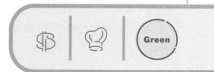

4 large Haas avocados, peeled and
    pitted
1 large plum tomato, diced
2 medium yellow tomatoes, diced
⅔ small Bermuda onion, diced

2 chives, finely chopped
½ cup finely chopped fresh cilantro
1½ tablespoons lemon juice
12 turns of red peppercorns
Salt and pepper to taste

Combine all ingredients in a large bowl and mix/smash together. Salt and pepper generously.

Joe's Black Bean Spread

Joe Rowley   SERVES 10 TO 12

Joe: *"Wow, if I could get this in a jar, I'd buy it by the case," said a friend on the evening I invented this stuff. That sounded enough like an endorsement to convince me to write it down. Like so many good food combinations, this one was made up on the spur of the moment. Some friends had gathered at our studio for a drink after work, and, of course, there was nothing readily available to snack on. We had a loaf of Italian sourdough bread, some black beans, red bell peppers, a couple of jalapeño and serrano peppers, and the usual things like olive oil, herbs, et cetera. So I thought, Hmmm, why not make a spread, grill the bread, and let everyone snack away.*

Marilu: *This is very easy to make and easy to store if you can keep it around that long. It has a unique flavor and is great to nibble on with guests, while cooking.*

Tasters' comments: *"I could wash my face in this, it tastes so good!"*

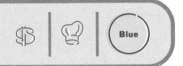

Three 30-ounce cans black beans

1 cup fresh cilantro

6 cloves garlic

3 jalapeño peppers

2 serrano peppers

½ medium red onion

¼ teaspoon dried chilies arbol flakes

1 teaspoon ground cumin

Extra-virgin olive oil as needed

1 tablespoon chopped fresh oregano

1 tablespoon chopped fresh thyme

Juice of 1 lime

Salt and pepper

2 red bell peppers

1 sourdough baguette

Drain the black beans, but keep some of the liquid. Pick the leaves from a bunch of cilantro, wash them, and spin them dry with a salad spinner. Peel and smash the garlic. Remove the seeds and ribs from the jalapeño and serrano peppers. Coarsely chop the chile peppers and the red onion. In a food processor with a steel blade, puree two cans of drained beans (the third will be added whole later), the onion, jalapeños, serranos, chilies arbol, garlic, ¾ cup of the cilantro, cumin, 1 tablespoon of olive oil, oregano, thyme, lime juice, and salt and black pepper to taste.

The puree should have the consistency of a milk shake that you'd have to eat with a spoon. If it's too thick, add a little of the reserved bean liquid and process some more. (But be careful. Remember, this is a spread, not soup.) If it's not spicy enough, add more chilies arbol. When it's all just right, put the puree into a large bowl.

Remove seeds and ribs from the red bell peppers, cut them into chunks, and use the food processor to finely chop. Add them and the reserved whole beans to the bean puree and mix thoroughly. Finely chop the remaining cilantro and garnish the top with it.

Pour some olive oil into a shallow bowl. Cut the sourdough bread into ½-inch-thick rounds, dip one side in the oil, and place the oiled rounds under the broiler to toast.

Now comes the fun part. Put the toasted sourdough rounds on a serving plate next to the bowl of bean spread and watch your friends make it disappear.

Tuscan White Bean Dip

Elizabeth Carney

Marilu: *The perfect dish when you're in a hurry to set out something quick, easy, and delicious. Can be served with veggies or pita bread. Great starter if your entree is miscombined.*

Tasters' comments: *"Hands down a winner."*

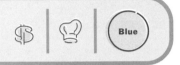

2 cans white beans
1 raw garlic clove, or 2 roasted garlic
 cloves
½ teaspoon salt

½ teaspoon vegetable bouillon
6 chives
Leaves from 4 sprigs rosemary
1 tablespoon olive oil

Puree all ingredients together in food processor.

Smoked Salmon Spread

Ruth A. Johnson

Ruth: This is an adaptation of a recipe I discovered during my stay in Paris.

Marilu: This great party spread is wonderful with cucumber, celery, and carrots. With tomato and onion on a bagel, it fooled my deli-loving mother-in-law.

Tasters' comments: "Perfect spread for bagels and toast points."

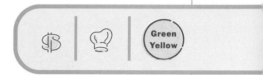

12 ounces smoked salmon

1 cup soy cream cheese

2 tablespoons prepared horseradish

1 teaspoon lemon juice

½ cup minced fresh parsley

Place salmon in a medium bowl and separate into flakes. Add remaining ingredients (except parsley) and stir until of spreading consistency. Shape mixture into a log shape and roll in parsley to coat. Refrigerate for several hours or overnight.

TV Tray-l Mix

Erin Reid

Erin: I have been thinking of trying a new recipe for a trail mix snack. I saw it on the side of a Chex box, but of course theirs has butter in it. Here is my version.

Marilu: A great answer to a snack. Kids love it. Surprise! We served it at a sports party and it disappeared before the pretzels.

Tasters' comments: "Can we have it in our lunch box?" "Great for the car."

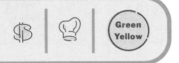

3 cups Shredded Spoonfuls
3 cups Multi-Grain Oatios
1 cup pretzels

1 cup raisins
1 cup banana chips or soy nuts
1 cup carob chips

Mix together in a Ziploc bag. If you are a big food combiner, you may want to omit the raisins, because I think that is a no-no.

Healthy Trail Mix

Darlene Reeves

Marilu: This easy-to-keep snack is great for school lunches. Kids find it fun to eat. After school they'll reach for it because it's easy to keep in the cupboard.

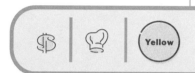

½ pound or 1 cup sunflower seeds

½ pound or 1 cup pumpkin seeds

½ pound or 1 cup raisins

½ pound almonds

½ pound carob chips (optional)

I usually mix 1 cup of each except for the carob chips; I add those sparingly. I hope you can use this, for it is a healthy snack for children. You can adjust the amounts according to what you like.

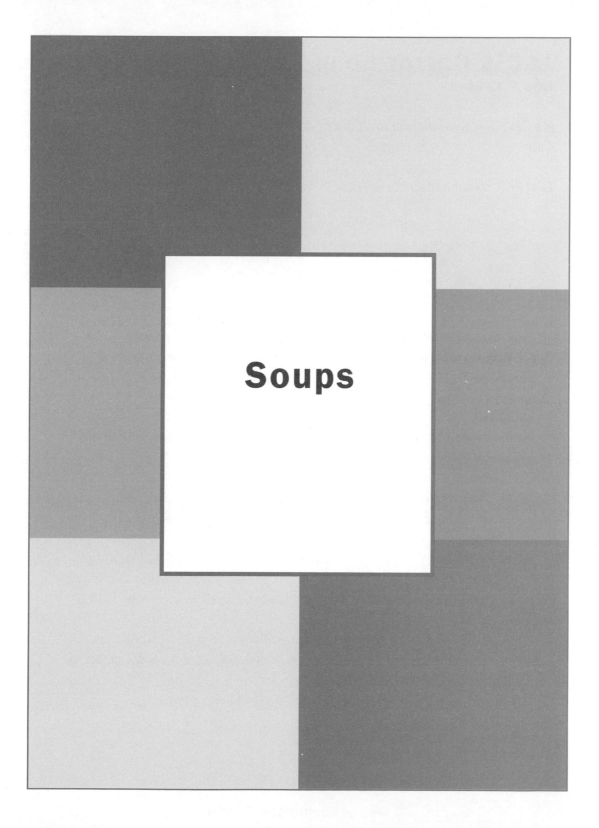

Soups

JAC's Carrot Soup

Julie A. Cirksena   SERVES 8

Marilu: This is one of those soups that we made over and over again. It's got a spicy sweet flavor.

Tasters' comments: "It's fantastic." "A real winner."

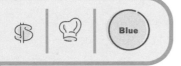

2 cups vegetable broth
6 medium carrots, washed and
   shredded
3 medium potatoes, peeled and
   shredded
1 medium onion, chopped
½ teaspoon salt

1 teaspoon ground pepper
½ tablespoon Italian seasoning
¼ teaspoon nutmeg
½ cup soy milk
¼ cup rice milk
½ stick soy margarine, softened

Combine 2 cups of water, the broth, carrots, potatoes, onion, salt, and pepper in a large pot and bring to a boil over high heat. Reduce heat to low, cover, and simmer for 15 minutes, or until carrots and potatoes are tender.

Remove the pot from heat. Transfer the mixture to a blender, 1 to 2 cups at a time, and place the lid on the blender, leaving the top slightly ajar to allow steam to escape (very important tip!). Carefully blend the mixture at low speed until smooth.

Return the blended mixture to the pot and place on high heat. Add Italian seasoning and nutmeg and bring mixture to a boil. Stir in milks and margarine until blended and heat thoroughly.

Ladle the soup into individual serving bowls and serve hot.

Wild Mushroom Soup

Denise Barker   SERVES 6

Denise: This is a rather unusual, exotic-tasting soup.

Marilu: This soup dances off your tongue. Thumbs up all around.

Tasters' comments: "Absolutely perfect."

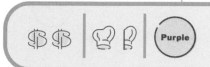

½ teaspoon sea salt

⅓ cup uncooked wild rice, well rinsed

2 tablespoons olive oil

3 medium cloves garlic, minced

1 medium onion, chopped

2 tablespoons chopped fresh thyme
   or 4 teaspoons dried

1 pound mixed mushrooms, such as
   shiitake, oyster, and cremini,
   chopped

6 cups vegetable broth

¼ teaspoon freshly ground white
   pepper

In a medium saucepan, bring 1 cup water and salt to a boil. Stir in wild rice and return to a boil. Reduce heat to low, cover, and simmer until tender, about 30 to 50 minutes. Drain and set aside.

Meanwhile, in a large saucepan, heat oil over medium-high heat. Add garlic, onion, and thyme and cook, stirring often, for 2 minutes. Add mushrooms, reduce heat to medium, and cook, stirring occasionally, until onion is tender, about 7 minutes. Add broth and bring to a boil. Reduce heat to low, cover, and simmer for 20 minutes. Transfer half of soup to blender and blend until almost pureed. Return to the saucepan and stir in wild rice and pepper. Return to a simmer over medium high heat. Cover, reduce heat to low, and simmer 10 minutes. Adjust seasoning to taste.

Homemade Vegetable Stock

Marilu: *This rewarding piece of excellence is a great starter for many of our sauces and soups.*

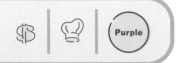

2 medium unpeeled russet potatoes,
    coarsely chopped

2 medium yellow onions, diced

1 rib celery, chopped

½ pound mushrooms

2 cups assorted vegetables, chopped
    (your choice, use whatever is left-
    over in the fridge)

5 cloves garlic, chopped

2 bay leaves

3 teaspoons fresh rosemary

3 teaspoons fresh basil

1 teaspoon fresh thyme

½ teaspoon peppercorns

¾ teaspoon salt

Put 10 cups of water in a large stockpot over medium-high heat. Add all the vegetables, garlic, herbs, peppercorns, and salt and bring to a boil. Reduce heat to low and simmer, uncovered, 45 minutes. Turn off heat and allow the mixture to steep for an additional 15 to 30 minutes before straining into a separate pot or large bowl. Any stock you do not use immediately may be stored for several days in the refrigerator or for several months in the freezer.

Country Vegetable Soup

SERVES 8

Marilu: It's so easy to make and because you don't have to cook it for a very long time, it's fresh and fast to the table. Tastes great the next day.

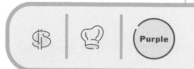

2 tablespoons vegetable concentrate (Organic Gourmet Instant Soup N' Stock or any healthy vegetable concentrate)

1 medium yellow onion, chopped

2 tablespoons chopped parsley

2 cups chopped celery

2 cups chopped carrots

2 cups potatoes, peeled and cut into bite-size chunks

2 cups cabbage

1 cup frozen peas

1 cup frozen green beans

Add vegetable concentrate to 2½ quarts hot water, or adjust amount of water to taste. Add onion, parsley, celery, carrots, and potatoes and cook soup on low heat for 10 to 15 minutes. Last, add cabbage, frozen peas, and frozen green beans. Continue cooking about 5 minutes or until potatoes are soft. Never overcook the vegetables.

Cilantro Corn Chowder

SERVES 8

Marilu: This fresh and healthy-tasting chowder really has a hearty flavor without being too filling.

Tasters' comments: "You can really taste all of the flavors." "Excellent."

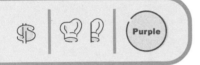

1 tablespoon olive oil

1½ cups red onion, chopped

1 cup diced carrot

1½ cups diced yellow bell pepper

1½ cups diced red bell pepper

4 cups potatoes, peeled and cubed

2 tablespoons vegetable soup concentrate

3 cups frozen or fresh corn kernels

3 tablespoons fresh cilantro

2 tablespoons chopped chives

Salt and pepper to taste

1 avocado, sliced (optional)

Put olive oil in a large soup pot. Add onion, carrot, and bell peppers and sauté until the vegetables soften, 4 to 6 minutes. Add potatoes and mix well into the vegetable mixture. Sauté an additional 7 to 8 minutes. Add 7½ cups water and bring to a boil. Cover and simmer over medium-low heat for 15 minutes.

Remove ½ cup of broth and dissolve soup concentrate into it. Add this to soup and mix well. Cook soup an additional 3 minutes, stirring continuously. Remove ⅓ of the soup with lots of vegetables in it and set aside. Blend remaining ⅔ of the soup until smooth in a blender or food processor. Stir in reserved soup, corn, cilantro, and chives. (If you want to thicken the soup up just a bit more, blend a few more of the whole vegetables from soup with 1 cup of corn.)

Bring soup to a low boil, stirring frequently, and simmer for 10 minutes on low heat, continuing to stir so that soup doesn't stick to bottom. Season to taste.

Serve with sliced avocado on top if desired.

Cream of Watercress Soup

Elizabeth Carney

SERVES 4

Marilu: This was a favorite of mine before I gave up dairy, so I'm thrilled that this flavor has come back into my life. Without the dairy, of course.

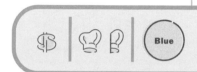

4 tablespoons soy butter

2 cups finely chopped yellow onions

½ cup minced shallots

3 cups vegetable stock plus more as
    needed

1 medium potato, peeled and diced

4 bunches watercress

1 cup soy cream

Salt and freshly ground black pepper
    to taste

Ground nutmeg and cayenne pepper
    to taste

Melt the soy butter in a heavy pot. Add the onions and shallots and cook, covered, over low heat until tender and lightly colored, about 25 minutes.

Add 3 cups vegetable stock and the potato, bring to a boil, reduce heat, and simmer, partially covered, until potato is very tender, about 20 minutes.

Meanwhile, remove the leaves and tender stems from the watercress and rinse thoroughly. When potato is tender, add watercress to the pot, cover, remove from heat, and let stand for 5 minutes.

Pour soup through a strainer, reserving liquid, and transfer the solids to the bowl of a food processor fitted with a steel blade, or use a food mill fitted with the medium disc. Add 1 cup of the cooking stock and process until smooth.

Return puree to the pot, stir in the soy cream, and add additional stock, ½ to 1 cup, until soup is of the desired consistency.

Set over medium heat, season to taste with salt, pepper, nutmeg, and cayenne, and simmer just until heated through. Serve immediately.

Cream of Tomato Soup

Tasters' comments: *"You can really taste the flavor of the fresh tomatoes." "You'll never eat canned again."*

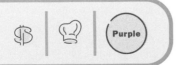

2¼ pounds (4 large) vine-ripened tomatoes

¼ cup extra-virgin olive oil, plus more for drizzling

4 large cloves garlic, bruised

Handful of fresh basil leaves, torn into small pieces (about 3 tablespoons)

4 cups vegetable broth

½ pound stale wheat bread, still soft enough to be torn, shredded

1¼ teaspoon Bragg Liquid Aminos

Freshly ground black or white pepper

In a saucepan, bring to boil enough water to cover the tomatoes. Plunge the tomatoes into the boiling water for 30 seconds. Remove them promptly and place them under cold running water. Using a paring knife, peel off the skins. Cut the tomatoes in half and remove the seeds; dice the tomatoes.

In a saucepan over medium-high heat, warm ¼ cup oil and garlic together. Sauté gently until the garlic is lightly golden, about 4 minutes. Add the tomatoes and about 2 tablespoons of the basil. Simmer over medium-low heat until the tomatoes thicken, about 20 minutes. Add the broth and bring to a boil. Add the bread and toss all the ingredients together. Continue to cook just until heated through and the bread absorbs the liquid completely. Remove the garlic cloves (don't throw them away, as they can be spread onto bread). Add the Bragg's and pepper to taste.

Ladle into individual serving bowls. Divide the remaining 1 tablespoon or so of basil among the bowls, sprinkling it on top, and drizzle with additional olive oil.

Cream of Broccoli Soup

MaryAnn Hennings   MAKES 8 CUPS, SERVES 6

Marilu: This flavor is so vivid, it tastes like puree of broccoli. It is very fresh and delicious.

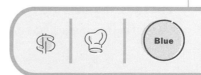

1½ pounds broccoli

2 tablespoons extra-virgin olive oil

1 tablespoon soy margarine

1 tablespoon minced garlic

1 cup diced onion (¼-inch dice)

½ cup diced celery (¼-inch dice)

Salt and freshly ground pepper

2 teaspoons finely chopped fresh
   thyme

5 cups "No" chicken stock (made by
   Imagine Foods) or vegetarian
   "chicken" stock

2 cups packed spinach

2 teaspoons freshly grated lemon
   zest

1 cup soy cream

1 tablespoon Bragg Liquid Aminos

Cut the broccoli florets from the stems. Peel the tough outer skin from the stems and trim off the fibrous ends. Cut the stems lengthwise into slices about ½ inch thick and then crosswise into ½-inch pieces.

Heat the olive oil and soy margarine in a soup pot over medium-high heat until hot. Add the garlic and cook until light brown. Add the onion and celery, lower the heat to medium, and season with salt. Cook the vegetables slowly until tender, about 10 minutes. Regulate the heat so the vegetables cook without taking on color.

Add the thyme and stir. Add the broccoli stems, stock, and salt and pepper to taste and bring to a boil. Cook, uncovered, for about 3 minutes. Add the florets and continue to cook until very tender, about 7 minutes more. Stir in the spinach and lemon zest. The spinach will wilt into the soup. Puree the soup in a blender in small batches. (The soup can be made to this point, covered, and refrigerated for up to 1 day or frozen for up to 1 month.)

Return the soup to the pan and reheat over gentle heat. Stir in the cream. Taste and adjust the seasoning with salt, pepper, and Bragg's. Ladle into warm bowls.

Creamy Daikon Soup

Elizabeth Carney

SERVES 6 TO 8

Marilu: This is one of my favorite recipes in this book. Enjoy!

Tasters' comments: "Creamy and delicious unusual flavor is a winner on rainy days." "One of my top three soups ever!"

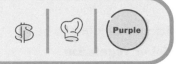

3 tablespoons soy margarine
2 cups finely chopped yellow onion
½ cup minced shallots
4 cups vegetable stock

2 long, large daikon radishes (cut in small pieces)
Salt and pepper to taste

Melt soy margarine in a heavy pot. Add onions and shallots and cook, covered, over low heat until tender.

Add vegetable stock and daikon radishes and bring to a boil. Reduce heat and simmer until daikon is tender, about 20 minutes.

Pour soup through a strainer. Reserve the liquid and transfer the solids to a blender or food processor. Puree, adding the reserved broth.

Return soup to pot and add more broth or water until you have reached desired consistency. Season to taste with salt and pepper.

Potato Leek Soup

SERVES 8

Marilu: This light-tasting soup is a great starter or a main course with bread.

Tasters' comments: "Scrumptious."

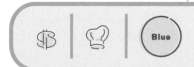

2 tablespoons soy margarine
1 large bunch leeks, julienned
6 new red potatoes, peeled and
    cubed
6 cups vegetable stock

¾ cup soy milk
½ teaspoon ground nutmeg
½ teaspoon black pepper
Salt
Fresh chives for garnish

Melt the margarine in a large stockpot over medium-low heat and add the leeks. Cook, covered, for about 15 minutes, or until they have softened.

Raise the heat to high, add the potatoes and stock, and bring to a boil. Reduce heat to low and cook, partially covered, about 25 minutes, or until the potatoes are tender.

Transfer the solids to a blender or food processor fitted with a steel blade and gradually add broth, pulsing until just pureed. Return the puree to the pot. Do not overheat or the potatoes will become elastic. Add soy milk, nutmeg, black pepper, and salt to taste. Serve garnished with chives.

Joanna's Gazpacho

Joanna Gleason

Marilu: My friend Joanna is a fabulous cook. Every time I go to her house I'm hoping she'll make this soup.

Tasters' comments: "Reminds me of summer evenings in Chicago." "This cold soup dropped me right on Logan Boulevard, singing songs of the seventies."

2 yellow or Vidalia onions

2 green peppers, seeded and
   chopped fine (not mushy)

2 red or orange or yellow peppers,
   seeded and chopped

2 large cucumbers, peeled, seeded,
   and chopped

½ cup olive oil

½ cup red wine vinegar

1½ cups tomato juice

Pinch of cayenne

3 tablespoons chopped dill

3 tablespoons chopped cilantro
   (optional)

4 small slices of avocado (optional)

Chop all vegetables, put in large bowl or tureen. Whisk oil, vinegar, and tomato juice together, adding cayenne, dill, and cilantro. Pour over vegetables, mix gently. Chill 3 hours or more, covered. Serve plain, or with small slice of avocado on top.

Chicago Diner's Miso Soup

SERVES 8

Chicago Diner: In fall and winter, use dark mugi barley miso. We have a friend who makes great misos in Wisconsin. In spring and summer, we use sweet white or yellow miso.

Marilu: My favorite soup from one of my favorite restaurants! I specifically asked for this when I started to write this book. It's a great winter soup as is.

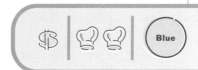

**5 cups filtered water or vegetable
  stock**
1 medium onion, sliced
2 cups sliced green cabbage
2 small carrots, julienned

½ cup miso
2 tablespoons mirin or rice wine
2 teaspoons minced ginger
2 tablespoons tamari or soy sauce

Bring water or vegetable stock to boil. Add sliced vegetables and cook 3 to 5 minutes to your liking, crunchy or soft. Turn off heat.

In a bowl, whisk the miso, mirin, ginger, and tamari with some hot broth. Add back to soup. You can adjust to your taste by adding more miso or ginger or soy sauce.

Note: Use less miso in warmer weather. Add Asian vegetables, sea vegetables (arame, dulse, et cetera), shiitake mushrooms, or firm tofu cubes for a heartier soup. Sesame oil is also a nice flavor addition.

Savory Squash Soup

Evelyn Kita

SERVES 8 TO 10

Marilu: This soup is light but effectively delicious. A hearty stew quality that delivers like a whole meal.

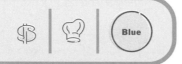

1 medium squash (most any kind, but spaghetti works well), cut into cubes

3 tablespoons olive oil

1 medium onion, diced

4 cups water

4 cups chicken or vegetable broth

½ cup red lentils

½ cup green lentils

½ cup finely chopped celery

4 cloves garlic, minced

½ teaspoon mild curry

½ teaspoon coriander

3 or 4 medium tomatoes, skinned and diced

¼ cup fresh parsley

1 to 3 tablespoons red wine or red wine vinegar to taste

Salt and pepper to taste

In a frying pan over medium heat, sauté squash in 2 tablespoons olive oil until slightly caramelized.

In another pan over medium heat, cook onion in 1 tablespoon olive oil until caramelized.

Place water and broth in large pot and add lentils and celery. Cook over low heat until lentils are soft, 10 to 15 minutes. Add garlic, spices, squash, and onions. Cook for 10 to 15 minutes more, then add tomatoes and parsley.

During the last 5 minutes of cooking, add red wine and salt and pepper to taste. Simmer 5 minutes more. Happy eating.

Tip: To peel a tomato, boil a pot of water. Stick a fork in the tomato and immerse it for five seconds. You will be amazed at how easily the peel comes off.

Lusty Lentil Soup

Ruth E. Stoll

Marilu: *Ruth Stoll is the mother of a good friend of mine, Mindy Paige Davis. She just happened to send to my website this very easy-to-make soup that is rich in flavor and very low fat. It is surprisingly filling.*

Tasters' comments: *"I love the beans."*

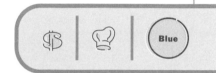

2 cups lentils

8 ounces (or more) sliced mushrooms

1 teaspoon olive oil

8 cups filtered water

2 or 3 vegetable bouillon cubes

3 medium carrots, sliced thin

2 or 3 medium onions, chopped

1 or 2 celery ribs, chopped

1 teaspoon basil

½ teaspoon marjoram

½ teaspoon salt (or to taste)

2 or 3 pieces kombu seaweed

Sort and rinse lentils. Sauté mushrooms in olive oil. Place lentils, sautéed mushrooms, and remaining ingredients in a large pot. Bring to a boil. Reduce heat and simmer 1 to 1½ hours.

Black Bean Soup

Marilu: Let's see, how shall I describe this . . . I'll just give you some of the quotes. It truly was a hit with everyone.

Tasters' comments: "I'm in heaven when I taste this." "Wonderful."

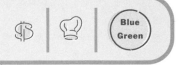

Four 15-ounce cans black beans

8 cups water or vegetable broth

2 carrots, diced

1 small red onion, chopped

4 cloves garlic, finely chopped or pressed

1 slice fresh ginger, the size of a quarter, finely chopped

2½ teaspoons chili powder

2 teaspoons ground cumin

Optional Toppings

Lime quarters

Chopped fresh cilantro

Chopped fresh basil

Chopped scallions

Soy sour cream

Place all the ingredients (except the toppings) in a heavy-bottomed 8-quart stockpot and bring to a gentle boil. Reduce heat to low and cook, partially covered, for 2 to 4 hours, depending upon consistency desired.

If you want a pureed soup or partially pureed soup, simply place at least half of the soup, in batches, in a blender or food processor fitted with a steel blade and blend until smooth.

Just prior to serving, if desired, squeeze the juice of ¼ lime on each serving and garnish with cilantro, basil, scallions, and soy sour cream.

Rob's Riot Soup

Robert Lieberman

Marilu: This soup was named after the time my husband made a huge pot of it for the neighbors during the L.A. riots. It's a surefire winner, no matter what's going on in your city.

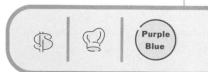

1 tablespoon olive oil
2 cups diced white onions
1½ cups diced celery
½ cup diced carrot
4 cups peeled and cubed potatoes
(½-inch cubes)

¼ teaspoon ground sage
8 cups water
2 tablespoons light miso or vegetable
broth
3 cups fresh or frozen corn kernels
1 scallion, chopped

In a large soup pot, add oil, onions, celery, and carrot and sauté over medium heat until vegetables begin to soften, approximately 3 to 5 minutes. Add potatoes and sage. Mix well and sauté an additional 3 minutes. Add water, bring to a boil, cover, and simmer over medium-low heat for 10 to 15 minutes, or until potatoes are tender, but not mushy.

Remove ½ cup of broth and add miso to it. Dissolve and then add to soup and mix well. Cook an additional minute, stirring occasionally.

Remove ⅓ of the soup with lots of vegetables in it and set aside. Blend remaining ⅔ of the soup until smooth with a hand blender or food processor. Stir in reserved soup, corn, and scallion.

Bring soup to a low boil, stirring frequently, and simmer for 10 minutes on low heat, continuing to stir so soup does not stick to the bottom.

Swiss Chard and Country Bean Soup

SERVES 4 TO 6

Marilu: *This is a very hearty pasta soup. It's filling, but doesn't make me feel stuffed. It has a nice balance of flavors.*

Blue Green

½ pound dried white beans (about 1¼ cups)

½ small onion

½ carrot

½ celery stalk

1 bay leaf

4 cups vegetable stock

Salt and freshly ground pepper

½ pound dried tubbetini or other medium-size pasta shape

½ cup extra-virgin olive oil

2 tablespoons thinly sliced garlic

½ teaspoon red pepper flakes

1 cup roughly chopped chard stems

4 cups roughly chopped chard greens, still wet from rinsing

1 tablespoon Bragg Liquid Aminos

¾ teaspoon finely chopped rosemary

2 tablespoons finely chopped flat-leaf parsley

½ cup freshly grated soy Parmesan

Pick over the beans to remove any small stones. Rinse and put in a small saucepan, add water to cover, and place over high heat. As soon as the beans begin to boil, remove from heat and let cool for about 1 hour.

Drain the soaked beans, rinse, and return to the pan with the onion, carrot, celery, and bay leaf. Add the vegetable stock and bring to a boil over high heat. Reduce heat to low, cover loosely, and simmer until beans are tender, 45 to 60 minutes. Add salt and pepper to taste only during the last half of cooking time. (Salting too early toughens the skins of the beans and lengthens cooking time.) Add more water if the beans absorb all the liquid before they cook through, but don't drown them. When the beans are cooked, drain, reserving the cooking liquid, and discard the onion, carrot, celery, and bay leaf.

Bring a large pot of water to a boil. Add salt and pasta and cook until al dente, about 12 minutes. Drain, refresh quickly under cool running water, and toss with about 1 tablespoon of the olive oil. Set aside.

Heat 2 tablespoons of the olive oil in a large sauté pan over medium heat until hot. Add the garlic and sauté briefly until light brown. Add the red pepper flakes, stir, and add the chard stems. Sauté for about 2 minutes. Add the chard, season with salt and pepper to taste, and cook until wilted, about 3 minutes. Add Bragg's and 3 cups of the reserved bean broth (add water to make up the amount, if necessary), bring to a simmer, and cook until the chard is tender, about 3 more minutes.

Add the beans and rosemary and cook until the beans are heated through. Add the pasta and continue to cook until heated through. Taste for salt and pepper and stir in the parsley. Pass the soy Parmesan and the remaining olive oil at the table.

Minestrone

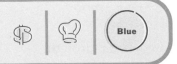

SERVES 8 TO 10

Marilu: This clean and simple minestrone has an old-world Italian flavor. It's like something from a café in Rome.

3 tablespoons extra-virgin olive oil, plus additional olive oil for the table

1 large carrot, scraped and diced

1 large onion, chopped coarsely

1 potato, peeled and diced

1 large celery stalk, thinly sliced, plus the leaves, chopped

¾ pound butternut squash, diced (1½ cups)

3 canned plum tomatoes, seeded and chopped, plus ¼ cup of their juices

2 teaspoons plus 3 tablespoons chopped fresh rosemary, or 1 teaspoon plus 2 tablespoons dried rosemary

6 tablespoons finely chopped fresh Italian parsley leaves and stems

½ pound green cabbage, finely shredded (about 1½ cups)

2 cups soaked and drained dried pinto beans (If you like, 1 cup dried cannellini beans can be substituted for the pinto beans)

3 quarts (12 cups) water

2 tablespoons salt, or to taste

Plenty of freshly ground black pepper

¼ pound green beans, cut into 1-inch lengths (about 1 cup)

2 small zucchini, cut crosswise into slices ½ inch thick

1½ cups cauliflower florets

1 cup conchigliette ("little shells") or ditalini ("little thimbles") pasta

4 large cloves garlic, finely chopped

Freshly grated soy Parmesan

In a large pot, combine the 3 tablespoons oil, carrot, onion, potato, celery and leaves, and squash. Sauté over medium heat for about 5 minutes, or until a little tender, stirring occasionally. Add the tomatoes with their juices, 2 teaspoons rosemary, 3 tablespoons parsley, cabbage, pinto beans, water, salt, and pepper. Cover the pot and bring to a boil over high heat. Immediately reduce the heat to medium-low, cover with the lid askew, and simmer for about 20 minutes.

Add the green beans, zucchini, cauliflower, and pasta; cook for 8 minutes. Stir in the garlic, 3 tablespoons rosemary, and 3 tablespoons parsley; if using canned beans, add them at this point. Continue cooking the soup, uncovered, over medium heat, until the pasta is not quite al dente (it will not remain so, since it soaks in the hot soup, so it is best to undercook it somewhat), about 8 minutes.

Serve the soup with grated soy Parmesan, a dribble of olive oil, and pepper to taste.

Rob's Ribollita

Robert Lieberman

Robert: *This is one of my favorite soups. It is particularly good if you can find fresh borlotti beans.* Ribollita *means "boiled again." It originally was a popular leftover dish; reheating it the next day and adding dry crusty bread gives this hearty soup its deep rich flavor. Ribollitas vary from region to region in Italy. I have seen this all the way from almost a consommé to a thick heavy bean soup. You can vary this by adding more or less broth and pureeing more or fewer of the beans. Although I love uniformly cut ingredients, for expediency I usually use the Cuisinart.*

Marilu: *My favorite of all of Rob's dishes. The most exquisite flavors in a perfect dish. Impossible not to have seconds. Make a lot, as it's even better the next day.*

Blue Green

2¾ cups (18 ounces) dried or fresh
   borlotti or cranberry beans
4 quarts water
1½ teaspoons salt
2 cloves garlic
2 tablespoons extra-virgin olive oil
1 large white onion (about 8 ounces),
   finely chopped
1 large carrot, peeled and cut into
   ¼-inch dice
2 stalks celery, trimmed and cut into
   ¼-inch dice
1 leek, white and tender green
   portion, cut into ¼-inch dice
1 medium-large tomato (about
   6 ounces), cut into ¼-inch dice

7 cups vegetable stock (canned or
   boxed, or made from powder or
   paste)
½ head green, black, or savoy cabbage (about 12 ounces), cut into
   1-inch chunks
2 teaspoons coarsely chopped sage
1 sprig fresh rosemary, or 1 teaspoon
   dried rosemary
½ teaspoon chopped fresh thyme
   leaves, or 1 teaspoon dried thyme
1 tablespoon coarsely chopped
   parsley leaves
6 slices dried pagnotta or any Italian
   bread, each about 1 inch thick
6 tablespoons grated soy Parmesan

In a large saucepan, place the dried beans and cold water to cover by about 1 inch, and soak at least 8 hours or overnight. Drain. Add the 4 quarts water and bring to a boil. Add 1 teaspoon of the salt and boil gently, with lid slightly ajar, for 1 hour. Drain and set aside.

Meanwhile, chop 1 of the garlic cloves. In a large heavy-bottomed saucepan over high heat, warm the olive oil. Add the chopped garlic and onion and sauté until the edges of the onion are slightly browned, about 5 minutes. Add the carrot, celery, leek, and tomato and sauté until the onion begins to soften and the tomato turns pale, about 5 minutes. Add the stock and the remaining ½ teaspoon salt, bring to a boil, and boil for about 30 minutes.

Using a fork, finely mash ¼ of the beans and set aside with the whole beans. Once the soup has boiled for 30 minutes, add the whole and mashed beans, cabbage, sage, rosemary, thyme, and parsley to the soup, reduce the heat to medium, and boil gently for 30 minutes. (The mashed beans will help to thicken the soup.)

If you do not have day-old bread as an option, preheat oven to 450 degrees. Prepare the bread slices. Lightly bruise the remaining garlic clove and rub it over both sides of each bread slice. Arrange the slices on a baking sheet and place on the lowest rack in the preheated oven. When the bottoms begin to toast, after 8 to 10 minutes, flip the slices over and toast an additional 2 minutes.

To serve, place a bread slice in the bottom of each individual bowl. (Depending upon the size and shape of your bowl, you may need to cut the slices so that they fit.) Ladle the soup over the bread and then sprinkle a tablespoon of the soy Parmesan over the top of each serving.

Another, easier way of serving is to take the bread and put it directly into the pot of soup, allowing the slices to partially fall apart, thickening the soup even more.

This soup is even better reheated the next day and progressively gets better upon every reheating.

Note: Dried beans should be put in a bowl, covered with water and allowed to soak overnight. You can use canned beans and add to the recipe at the same point you would add the prepared dried beans. You can substitute great Northern beans or any available bean, but the flavor will vary.

Cioppino

Elizabeth George

Tasters' comments: *"This is a great main-course soup." "This is a nice cold-weather soup." "There's something peasant-like and romantic about it."*

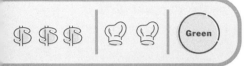

1 sea bass or striped bass	1 red bell pepper
1 monkfish	½ cup olive oil
1 pound shrimp	1 large onion, chopped
1 quart clams or mussels	2 cloves garlic, chopped
½ pound baby scallops (optional)	3 tablespoons chopped parsley
¼ pound dried mushrooms (Italian variety)	⅓ cup tomato puree
	1 pint red wine
3 or 4 tomatoes	Salt and pepper to taste

Cut the raw fish into serving-size pieces. Shell the shrimp, leaving the tails intact. Clean and steam the clams or mussels and save the liquid. Soak the mushrooms in cold water. Peel and chop the tomatoes and chop the bell pepper.

Place the olive oil in a deep pot, and when it is hot add the onion, garlic, parsley, mushrooms, and bell pepper and cook for 3 minutes. Next add the tomatoes and the puree, the wine, and the liquid from the clams or mussels. Salt and pepper to taste, cover, and simmer for 30 minutes. Add the cut-up fish and the shellfish, and cook until done.

Salads

Japanese Baby Green Salad

Marilu: *This Asian-inspired dressing really wakes up traditional salad greens.*

Tasters' comments: *"What a nice change from an Italian dressing." "Great salad with fish." "So yummy."*

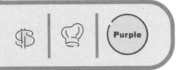

2 cups mixed baby greens

1 teaspoon Sucanat

¾ tablespoon white wine vinegar

¼ teaspoon sea salt

¼ teaspoon fresh ground pepper

2 tablespoons extra-virgin olive oil

Wash and dry the greens very well. In a bowl, whisk together Sucanat, vinegar, salt, and pepper. Add oil by drizzling it in. Toss the dressing and lettuce together so there is a fine coat of dressing covering all of the greens.

Tomato Onion Salad

MaryAnn Hennings

SERVES 4

Marilu: *MaryAnn is a great friend whose talent as a cook is surpassed only by her talent as a hairdresser. Through the program, she has lost twenty-five pounds and gained cooking expertise. This dish is a winner with the whole team.*

Tasters' comments: *"This one gets an A++." "It has a perfect combination of flavors." "This is the perfect salad when you want to do food combining." "It's like restaurant eating."*

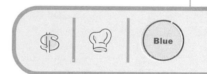

1 can great Northern beans

4 large or 5 small plum tomatoes, cut into bite-size chunks

1 small Maui onion, cut in half and sliced into thin strips

1 can anchovies in olive oil

2 tablespoons olive oil

2 tablespoons balsamic vinegar

2 to 3 teaspoons salt

Drain beans and add them to tomatoes and onions in a large bowl. Cut anchovies in half and separate. Add them to bowl; also add remaining oil from can. Add olive oil and vinegar. Stir together. Add salt to taste. Let marinate for at least an hour at room temperature.

Sun-Dried Tomato Salad with Basil Pesto Vinaigrette

Marilu: The basil vinaigrette works great on just regular greens too.

Tasters' comments: "Very hearty and flavorful."

   (Green)

Basil Pesto Vinaigrette

½ cup olive oil

½ cup packed fresh basil leaves

2 tablespoons balsamic vinegar

2 tablespoons lemon juice

2 tablespoons toasted pine nuts

12 cups mixed baby salad leaves

¼ cup coarsely chopped fresh basil

1 large red bell pepper, roasted, stemmed, seeded, and torn into long thin strips

1 large yellow bell pepper, roasted, stemmed, seeded, and torn into long thin strips

½ cup packed drained sun-dried tomatoes, cut into ½-inch pieces

½ cup toasted pine nuts

2 tablespoons finely chopped fresh chives

Make the basil pesto vinaigrette: Put all dressing ingredients into a food processor with the metal blade. Pulse the machine several times until mixture is coarsely chopped; then process continuously, stopping 2 or 3 times to scrape down sides of bowl, until dressing is smooth. Set aside.

Toss lettuce with fresh basil. Arrange mixture on salad plates. Garnish with peppers, sun-dried tomatoes, and pine nuts. Spoon dressing over salad. Garnish with chives.

Romaine and Fennel Salad

Marilu: *The fennel really breaks the traditional flavors found in a salad.*

Tasters' comments: *"This is very similar to a Caesar salad." "Excellent flavors."*

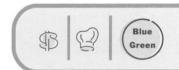

Salt
1 clove garlic, peeled
½ cup olive oil
1 tablespoon wine vinegar
1 tablespoon Nayonaise
Freshly ground black pepper

1 head romaine lettuce, torn into bite-size pieces
1 fennel bulb, cut in small thin strips
4 anchovy fillets, chopped
1 teaspoon capers
1 hard-cooked egg, sliced

Sprinkle the bottom of a salad bowl with salt and rub it with the garlic. Add the oil, vinegar, Nayonaise, and pepper. Stir with a wooden spoon until well blended.

Add the remaining ingredients and toss lightly with a fork and spoon.

What a Tomato Salad

Tasters' comments: *"This looks so pretty when the tomatoes are in season." "So flavorful!" "It allows your artistic side to shine."*

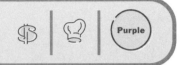

2 Italian plum tomatoes, cut in half

2 garden beefsteak tomatoes, sliced

8 small yellow pear tomatoes, sliced
  or left whole

Fresh basil

Fresh marjoram

Fresh black pepper

Have fun arranging the tomatoes. Cut them in slices, wedges, or halves. Arrange basil leaves in between and put a stem of marjoram lying over the top. Season with pepper. Serve plain or with a good herb-infused olive oil.

Two-Bean or Not Two-Bean Salad

SERVES 4

Marilu: This salad is a green bean lover's dream. It's a crunchy salad with a fresh, clean taste.

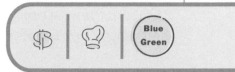

1 pound yellow and green beans

2 teaspoons pistachio nuts

1 teaspoon chopped chives

Dressing

¾ cup balsamic vinegar

½ cup olive oil

1 teaspoon Dijon mustard

Steam trimmed beans 2 to 4 minutes and rinse immediately under cold water to cool and refresh. Sprinkle pistachios and chives on top.

Whisk all dressing ingredients together and serve over top of salad.

Salad Greens with Fresh Cucumber Dressing

Joe Rowley   SERVES 4

Joe: This salad is so simple that it's almost silly to make a recipe for it. But whenever we've served it to guests, they almost always ask us to write it down. The only thing we've been able to figure out is that we've hit on a unique combination of greens, garnish, and dressing. It's a coming together of ingredients that's just right in both texture and flavor.

Tasters' comments: "I can't believe how this dressing hits all the right places on my palate." "I would recommend eating this salad after dinner, sort of European style, to clean the palate."

1 head red leaf lettuce

1 head green leaf lettuce

1 head Boston lettuce

4 plum tomatoes, sliced into
  ½-inch rounds

1 red onion, cut in half, then sliced
  thinly

1 cup chervil or parsley leaves

Dressing

1 tablespoon coarsely diced yellow
  onion

½ cucumber, peeled, seeded, and
  coarsely chopped

3 tablespoons white wine vinegar

½ cup extra-virgin olive oil

2 tablespoons fresh or 1 tablespoon
  dried dill or chives

Salt and pepper to taste

Peel off any bruised or damaged leaves from each head of lettuce. Cut the root ends off the heads of leaf lettuce 2 to 3 inches from the bottom. Cut the root end of the Boston lettuce much closer. When you do, you'll notice that the head has a rather hard, yellowish heart. Pull those pieces out, leaving only the tender greens. Cut or tear the lettuce leaves into bite-size pieces, wash in cold water, and spin them dry with your salad spinner. (If you don't have this device, go out right now and buy one. You'll thank us for many years.)

Toss all three types of lettuce together in a large bowl so they are all mixed together.

Put the dressing ingredients into a blender or food processor and blend for a short time. The vegetables will puree and the mixture will emulsify and turn into magical stuff. Taste it. Add salt or pepper to taste.

Now you're ready to assemble the salad. However, do not put it all together until you're ready to serve it.

Toss the greens with the pureed dressing and put the portions on 4 plates. Arrange the tomato slices around the outer edge of the greens, lay 2 half rings of red onion on top of each, and sprinkle the chervil or parsley leaves on top.

Watercress Salad with Tomatoes and Toasted Pine Nuts

SERVES 4

Marilu: You could serve this at the end of a meal as a palate cleanser.

Tasters' comments: "Very clean flavor." "What a great beginning for a many-flavored meal."

2 bunches watercress

12 little yellow tomatoes

½ cup toasted pine nuts

Champagne Vinaigrette (page 296)

Divide watercress and tomatoes onto 4 plates. Dress with champagne vinaigrette. Top with pine nuts.

Red Bean Salad

Stephanie O'Driscoll

Marilu: This amazingly colorful salad reminds me of the Fourth of July. It has three of my favorite veggies with beans.

Tasters' comments: "The textures and flavors are immense."

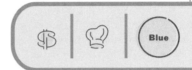

1 can kidney beans

4 or 5 thinly sliced radishes

2 cups shredded red cabbage

1 small yellow pepper, diced

1 small shallot, finely chopped

2 tablespoons chopped fresh parsley

Dressing

2 tablespoons red wine vinegar

1 tablespoon Dijon mustard

2 garlic cloves, minced

4 tablespoons olive oil

Pinch oregano (fresh or dried)

Salt and pepper to taste

Put salad ingredients together in a large bowl. Put dressing ingredients in a jar with screw-on lid and shake vigorously. Pour over salad and toss well.

Billy's Adzuki Bean Boom-Boom Salad

Billy Drake

SERVES 4

Marilu: *A salad as colorful and crazy as its chef. The perfect addition to any meal to make food combining effortless.*

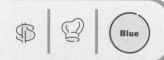

½ pound adzuki beans, washed,
    soaked, and strained

½ cup chopped red onions

2 cloves garlic, chopped

½ green bell pepper, chopped

½ red bell pepper, chopped

½ yellow bell pepper, chopped

Balsamic vinegar to drizzle

Salt and freshly ground pepper to
    taste

Juice of ½ lemon

Bring adzuki beans to boil for ½ hour, so they are firm but edible. Strain. Combine all other ingredients with the beans. Mix well and serve.

Shrimp and Chanterelle Salad

SERVES 4

Marilu: This great starter salad has a lightness to it. The shrimp and chanterelles work well together. They actually enhance each other's natural flavor.

Tasters' comments: "Elegant and delicious."

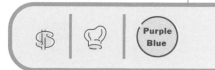

2 tablespoons salt

12 ounces large shrimp, peeled and deveined

8 ounces chanterelle mushrooms, cleaned and cut into bite-size pieces

Freshly ground pepper to taste

2 tablespoons extra-virgin olive oil

2 plum tomatoes, cut into wedges

In a large saucepan, bring to a boil 1 quart of water and the salt. Add shrimp and cook for 3 or 4 minutes. Remove them when they are almost fully cooked and let cool. Put the saucepan of water aside.

Season mushrooms with salt and pepper. Place olive oil in a skillet and heat on high, letting the oil get very hot. Carefully add mushrooms and sauté until soft (about 5 minutes). Remove them and let cool.

Season tomatoes with salt and pepper. In a bowl, put 2 teaspoons of water from the pot the shrimp was cooked in and a teaspoon of oil from the mushrooms and toss together with the shrimp, mushrooms, and tomatoes. Serve in small individual bowls or on plates.

Thai Shrimp and Asparagus Salad

Denise Barker

SERVES 4

Marilu: This is a great starter! The shrimp and asparagus balance each other nicely.

Tasters' comments: "It's so good." "I recommend it."

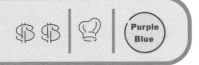

1½ pounds asparagus

1 tablespoon olive oil

1 teaspoon finely chopped ginger

1 clove garlic, finely chopped

8 ounces small to medium shrimp, peeled and deveined

1 tablespoon soy sauce

Sprinkle of hot sauce

Bring a pot of water to a boil and cook asparagus until just tender. Rinse in cold water. In a skillet, heat oil on medium and stir-sauté ginger for a minute, then add garlic and shrimp and cook until shrimp are pink. Stir in soy sauce and hot sauce. Remove from heat and allow to cool.

Joey's Tofu with Snapper Salad

Joseph Lieberman

SERVES 4

Marilu: My son Joey loves to cook and wanted to contribute to the book. We had ingredients left over from another recipe and this is what he put together. This has a great mixture of clean flavors. The snapper provides a firm hearty quality. It makes a great starter or lunchtime salad.

Tasters' comments: "I love this." "I can't believe a four-year-old could come up with this."

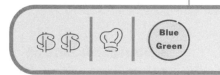

1 block firm tofu

3 scallions, chopped

½ bunch cilantro, chopped

½ bunch parsley, chopped

2 tablespoons sesame oil

2 tablespoons rice wine vinegar

2 tablespoons soy sauce

Juice of 1 lime

One 6- to 8-ounce fillet snapper

3 tablespoons extra-virgin olive oil

1 can Northern white beans

In a mixing bowl, mix together all ingredients except fish, olive oil, and beans. Mash with a potato masher so that all ingredients are well combined. Lightly brush the snapper with olive oil and grill 3 to 5 minutes on each side. Chop into squares and add to tofu mixture. Stir in white beans. This can be eaten alone or on top of a bed of greens.

Tuna and White Bean Salad

MaryAnn Hennings

SERVES 4

Marilu: This is a very impressive dish that's great for lunch or dinner. The white beans and the tuna really bring out each other's flavor.

3 tablespoons olive oil

1 leek, julienned, or ¼ Spanish
   onion, coarsely chopped

2 stalks celery, julienned

2 carrots, julienned

1 bay leaf

1 tablespoon fresh thyme

2 cups cooked white beans, canned
   or fresh

½ cup vegetable stock

2 tablespoons Bragg Liquid Aminos

1 fresh tuna steak (about 1 pound),
   1 to 1½ inches thick

Salt and pepper to taste

4 tablespoons balsamic vinegar

2 tomatoes, diced

¼ cup fresh chopped basil

Heat a large nonstick skillet over medium-low heat and add 2 tablespoons of olive oil. Add the leek or onion, celery, carrots, bay leaf, and thyme, and cook until the vegetables are soft, about 10 minutes. Add the beans, stock, and Bragg's and cook about 5 minutes, or until the beans are soft and heated through.

Remove the bay leaf. Scoop the vegetables and beans into a large serving dish.

Season the fish with salt and pepper. In the same pan, heat the remaining tablespoon of olive oil over medium-high heat and add the tuna. Cook for about 5 minutes per side or until desired doneness.

Cut the tuna into large chunks and arrange them on top of the bean mixture. Sprinkle with balsamic vinegar, tomatoes, and basil.

Smoked Salmon Salad with Cucumber and Pine Nuts

SERVES 4

Marilu: This salad is really wonderful and beautiful on the plate. Great color combination. This also works well as a light meal on its own. The pine nuts add an almost "cream cheese" quality to the salad.

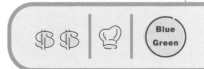

1 head red leaf lettuce
1 head green leaf lettuce
1 bunch fresh dill
Smoked salmon
Pickling cucumber rounds
Regular cucumber "batons"
Pine nuts (optional)

Dressing
¼ cup rice vinegar
¼ cup olive oil
Salt and pepper to taste

Assemble all salad ingredients in a bowl, add dressing ingredients, and toss.

Wild Rice and Soy Chicken Salad

MaryAnn Hennings

Marilu: This great lunch salad can be eaten cold or hot. For a change, you could make it without the soy chicken. It's a great dish to make with leftover rice.

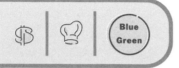

2 teaspoons olive oil

1 red onion, thinly sliced, or 1 bunch scallions, chopped

4 cups cooked wild rice

½ pound soy chicken strips

1 medium tomato, diced

2 tablespoons chopped fresh parsley

Dressing

8 sun-dried tomatoes, chopped

2 cloves garlic, chopped or pressed

3 tablespoons red wine vinegar

3 tablespoons balsamic vinegar

1 tablespoon Bragg Liquid Aminos

5 tablespoons olive oil

Heat a small nonstick skillet over medium heat and add the oil. When the oil is hot, add the onion or scallions and cook about 10 minutes, or until the onion is translucent. Set aside to cool.

Combine the wild rice, soy chicken, tomato, onion, and parsley in a large bowl and set aside.

Place all the dressing ingredients except the olive oil in a blender or food processor fitted with a steel blade and mix until well combined. While the motor is running, gradually add the olive oil.

Add the dressing to the rice mixture and serve either at room temperature or chilled.

Protein Entrées

Seared Tuna and Caramel Soy

SERVES 4

Marilu: The idea of "caramel soy" sounded so good to me, I had to have this recipe. It has a great Asian flavor. In a word, scrumptious.

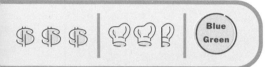

½ cup Sucanat
1 tablespoon water
½ cup soy sauce
2 garlic cloves
3 slices fresh ginger

8 tablespoons black and white
   sesame seeds
1 pound sushi-quality tuna
Salt
¼ cup peanut oil

In a small saucepan, add Sucanat and water and bring to a boil, stirring occasionally. When the mixture starts really cooking around the edges (about 5 minutes), remove from the heat. It's very hot and may splatter, so stand back and add the soy sauce. Stir in the garlic and ginger. Let it sit for about thirty minutes. Remove the ginger and garlic.

Place the sesame seeds on a plate. Wet fish on both sides, season with salt, and roll fish over sesame seeds until completely covered.

Heat oil in a large skillet over medium to high heat. Add fish and sear on both sides for about a minute or less, so that the sesame seeds are toasted and the fish is rare inside. Slice into ½-inch strips. Arrange on a plate and drizzle sauce over the top or serve sauce on the side in a little dipping bowl.

Sesame-Crusted Salmon

Marilu: This is a delicious dinner that will impress your friends. The best part is while you are finishing the fish in the oven, you have time to entertain your guests or to whip up a side dish.

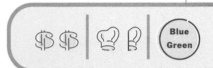

4 salmon fillets

Salt and pepper to taste

1 cup teriyaki sauce

½ cup sesame seeds

2 teaspoons soy margarine

2 teaspoons olive oil

In a shallow dish, season fish with salt and pepper. Marinate in teriyaki sauce for 20 minutes. Remove. Roll in sesame seeds.

Preheat oven to 275 degrees. In a large ovenproof skillet, sauté fish on all sides with soy margarine and olive oil over low heat for 5 minutes or until brown. To finish cooking, place fish in the oven for 5 to 7 minutes. Total cooking time should be 10 to 12 minutes.

Spicy Grilled Salmon

Marilu: *This spicy grilled salmon is easy to make and this recipe works well with sea bass and swordfish too. Also great on baby green salads for a lighter dinner or lunch.*

Tasters' comments: *"Salmon with a kick."*

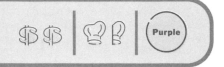

½ teaspoon salt

½ teaspoon cracked pepper

½ teaspoon garlic powder

¼ teaspoon cayenne pepper

¼ teaspoon paprika

4 salmon fillets

½ teaspoon olive oil

Mix all dry seasonings together. Rub salmon with olive oil and then coat with dry seasonings. Grill on very hot grill for 5 minutes on each side.

Olive's Grilled Marinated Tuna

Todd English from Olive's Restaurant

Marilu: *This is a very flavorful, simple dish. If you put the fish in the marinade in the morning, you'll have a quick weeknight dinner.*

Tasters' comments: *"What a great dish." "Fast, easy, and delicious." "I would recommend this highly."*

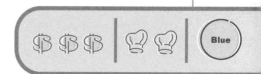

Marinade

¼ **cup olive oil**

2 **cloves garlic, finely chopped**

2 **teaspoons grated orange zest**

2 **tablespoons grated peeled fresh ginger**

½ **bunch fresh cilantro, leaves only, chopped**

Six 6- to 8-ounce very fresh bluefin or yellowfin tuna steaks, 1½ to 2 inches thick

1 **teaspoon kosher salt**

½ **teaspoon black pepper**

Olive's Citrus Aioli (page 292)

6 **fresh cilantro sprigs, for garnish**

Place the marinade ingredients in a large glass or ceramic bowl and stir to combine. Add the tuna, cover, and refrigerate for 4 hours or overnight.

Prepare the grill or preheat the broiler.

Sprinkle the tuna with the salt and pepper, place about 3 to 4 inches from the heat source, and grill or broil for 5 to 6 minutes per side; the tuna should still be rare.

Drizzle with the aioli and garnish with the cilantro sprigs.

Theresa's Fabulous Fish

Theresa Brown

SERVES 2

Marilu: A winner all around.

Tasters' comments: "She's right! It's fabulous." "Try it with snapper or cod. This is something to experiment with."

   Blue Green

2 to 3 tablespoons olive oil

2 leeks (white and pale green part only), well rinsed and sliced into long and thin strips

¼ cup lemon juice

3 tablespoons San-J teriyaki sauce

Up to 1 cup warm water

1 cup fresh shiitake mushrooms (stems removed), sliced into strips, or reconstituted dried shiitake mushrooms (stems removed; save the soaking water to flavor the sauce)

1 cup sun-dried tomatoes, sliced

One 1-pound fish fillet or steak, divided into 2 pieces

In a deep-sided skillet or pan, heat olive oil. Sauté the leeks until just tender. Add the lemon juice, teriyaki sauce, and ¼ to ½ cup of the warm water. Let the mixture heat up a bit, then add the mushrooms and sun-dried tomatoes and stir-sauté them briefly. Add the fish, turn down the heat to medium, and cover the pan, turning fish on its other side at least once. If most of the liquid it's poaching in seems to be drying up or cooking too fast, turn down heat slightly. Also, you can add more warm water as needed so it doesn't all cook away.

Divide fish onto plates, top with the leeks, mushrooms, and sun-dried tomatoes, and spoon sauce over it.

Baked Golden Trout

Elizabeth Carney

Marilu: You can try it with other small whole fish.

Tasters' comments: "Great flavor." "This is so simple, yet so good."
"Totally easy to prepare."

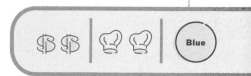

2 whole trout

Olive oil spray

1 bunch watercress

½ bunch Italian parsley

½ cup olive oil

3 to 6 sage leaves, cut

7 or 8 basil leaves, sliced thin

5 oregano leaves, chopped

2 green onions, chopped

¼ cup clam juice

⅓ cup white wine

2 tablespoons soy margarine

Preheat oven to 400 degrees. Clean fish and set aside.

Spray a baking dish with olive oil. Lay watercress and parsley in dish and place fish on top. In a sauté pan, simmer olive oil, sage, basil, oregano, onions, clam juice, and white wine for 3 to 5 minutes or until alcohol burns off. Add soy margarine. Whisk together. Pour mixture into belly of the fish and whatever remains onto the top of fish. Bake 10 minutes per inch of thickness.

Whole Roasted Fish with Fennel

SERVES 4

Marilu: This dish reminds me of the south of France. I love fish on the bone. It's so flaky, it melts on your tongue.

1 large fennel bulb, including stems and feathery leaves
¼ cup best-quality olive oil
1 shallot
2 garlic cloves, peeled and minced
Salt and freshly ground black pepper to taste
½ cup chopped Italian parsley

1 whole fish, 5 to 7 pounds before dressing, backbone removed, scaled, head and tail intact (striped bass or red snapper work best)
Juice of ½ lime
½ cup dry white wine or vermouth
Fresh watercress for garnish

Preheat oven to 400 degrees. Cut fennel bulb into slices and the slices into thin strips. Reserve stems and feathery leaves. Heat olive oil in a small skillet and sauté fennel strips, shallot, and half of the garlic, covered, until just tender, about 10 minutes. With a slotted spoon, transfer fennel to a bowl, season with salt and pepper to taste, and add the parsley. Reserve the oil.

Arrange the fish in an oiled shallow baking dish and spread it open. Lay the cooked fennel mixture down the center of the fish. Sprinkle with lime juice, close the fish, and tie it together in two or three places with kitchen twine.

Season the outside of the fish with salt and pepper and rub it with the remaining garlic clove. Pour reserved oil over the fish and lay reserved fennel stems and leaves on top. Pour white wine or vermouth into the pan.

Bake fish on middle rack of oven for 10 minutes per inch of thickness. Baste often with accumulated juices from the pan. Fish is done when flesh is opaque and flakes slightly when probed with a fork. Remove strings.

Serve at once surrounded with fresh watercress on a large serving platter.

Grilled Snapper

Marilu: This dish can be done with many different fillets. If it doesn't grill well, try broiling in a pan. It's simple and good, and also works well with bass, salmon, or chicken.

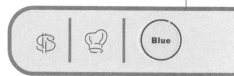

Marinade
Juice of 1 lime
1 ripe tomato
1 shallot, finely chopped
1 garlic clove, minced

1 teaspoon olive oil
½ cup white wine
Salt and pepper to taste

1 fresh red snapper fillet

Mix marinade ingredients together in a bowl. Soak the fish in marinade at room temperature for 20 to 30 minutes. Be careful not to overmarinate, because the lime juice cooks the fish like a ceviche. Grill 3 to 5 minutes each side.

Honey Teriyaki Cod

Elizabeth Carney

SERVES 1

Elizabeth Carney: Some stores will have a bottled teriyaki sauce with honey already mixed into it. If you can only find teriyaki, add 2 teaspoons honey to ½ cup teriyaki per fillet.

Marilu: This very simple Asian-influenced fish falls apart, it's so tender. Great fast meal for one.

Tasters' comments: "One of my favorites in the book."

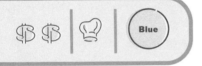

1 cod fillet
½ cup honey teriyaki sauce
Canola oil spray

Marinate the fish in the teriyaki sauce for 30 to 45 minutes at room temperature.

Spray a frying pan with canola oil and heat on high. Quickly sear the cod, turning it periodically, until it almost falls apart and it is golden brown.

Baked Salmon with Sun-Dried Tomato Crust

SERVES 4

Marilu: This salty-tasting fish is "alive with flavors." The spices and olives blend well with the sun-dried tomato crust.

Tasters' comments: "You'll be craving it the next day."

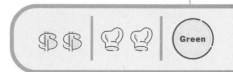

¼ cup chopped, pitted calamata olives

¼ cup chopped, pitted green olives

¼ cup chopped and drained oil-packed sun-dried tomatoes

3 garlic cloves

2 tablespoons soy margarine

1½ teaspoons fresh rosemary

2 teaspoons fresh thyme

6 teaspoons Dijon mustard

1 cup panko (a Japanese bread crumb) or very fine regular bread crumbs

Olive oil spray

Four 6-ounce salmon fillets

Preheat oven to 400 degrees. Mix black and green olives, sun-dried tomatoes, garlic, margarine, rosemary, and thyme in a medium bowl. Mix in 2 teaspoons of Dijon mustard, then panko. Spray a large baking sheet with olive oil. Place salmon fillets on prepared sheet. Spread 1 teaspoon of mustard over each. Pack one-fourth of panko mixture onto each mustard-coated fillet. Bake fillets until they are just opaque in center, about 12 minutes.

Baked Salmon with Tomatoes, Olives, and Capers

a tavola   SERVES 6

a t a v o l a : I brought the very best of Italian cooking back to my restaurant, a tavola, in the United States, after working as the chef of an Italian restaurant in Italy. A tavola has been re-creating classic Italian recipes in Chicago for five years, with a focus on the Italian use of fresh and simple ingredients.

This baked salmon recipe is an adaptation of Chef Ariel Leifer's mother's, which has been a Leifer household favorite since Ariel was a child.

M a r i l u : I personally requested this dish for the book because I enjoyed it so much when I ate at a tavola. Now it's your turn.

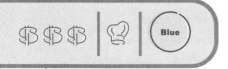

1 tablespoon minced garlic

½ cup diced red onion

3 tablespoons olive oil

¼ cup red wine

¼ cup white wine

6 tablespoons capers

½ tablespoon rosemary, chopped finely

⅛ teaspoon red pepper flakes

½ cup canned crushed tomatoes

12 pitted black olives

Six 6-ounce salmon fillets

Salt and freshly ground black pepper

6 tablespoons chopped parsley

In a saucepan on medium-low heat sauté the garlic and onion in the olive oil until the onion is translucent. Add all the remaining ingredients except the fish, salt and pepper, and parsley and simmer for 10 minutes.

Heat the oven to 500 degrees. Pour the sauce into a baking dish, lay the fillets in the sauce, and baste lightly with the sauce. Season with salt and pepper. Bake about 10 minutes, until fish is done. Sprinkle with parsley.

Miso-Glazed Sea Bass

Marilu: This has a great Asian flavor. A healthy, beautiful dinner.

Tasters' comments: *"This dish goes well with brown rice and steamed soybeans."*

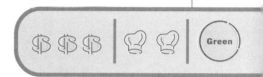

⅓ cup sake

⅓ cup mirin

⅓ cup light yellow miso

3 tablespoons Sucanat

2 tablespoons tamari

Four 6-ounce sea bass fillets

2 tablespoons chopped scallions

2 tablespoons chopped fresh basil

Mix the sake, mirin, miso, Sucanat, and tamari in a shallow baking dish. Add fish and turn it over to coat. Cover and refrigerate. Marinate for 2 to 6 hours. Preheat the broiler. Remove fish from marinade and place on a rimmed baking sheet with the broiler door slightly open. Broil the fish until just opaque in the center, about 6 minutes. Transfer to plate. Sprinkle with scallions and basil and serve.

Herb-Infused Whole Baked Fish

SERVES 4

Marilu: Make sure your guests know this fish has eyes. One of my favorite ways to eat fish.

Tasters' comments: "What a sweet flaky flavor." "This is easy to make, yet totally impressive."

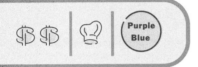

2 tablespoons olive oil	1 bunch rosemary
1 large yellow onion, chopped	½ cup white wine
1 whole fish (works well with striped bass, red snapper, or trout), cleaned	Olive oil spray
	1 clove garlic, minced
1 bunch marjoram	1 bunch parsley

In a sauté pan, combine the olive oil and onion. Cook until golden brown. Stuff the fish with half the marjoram, half the rosemary, and half the onion. Place in an oil-sprayed baking dish. Add white wine and garlic to the onion remaining in the pan and sauté on low heat for approximately 7 minutes or until alcohol is burned off. Pour this mixture over the fish and surround fish with the remaining marjoram and rosemary and the parsley. Cook at 400 degrees for 10 minutes per each inch of thickness.

Fan-Mail Flounder with Mustard

SERVES 4

Marilu: This very easy-to-make dish is excellent with a simple vegetable side dish.

Tasters' comments: "Really tasty." "Not what you would normally expect from a flounder."

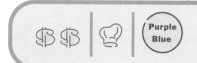

4 skinless and boneless flounder fillets (about 1½ pounds)
Freshly ground black pepper (7 turns
  of the pepper mill)

1½ tablespoons olive oil
2½ tablespoons Dijon mustard
2 tablespoons chopped chives
½ lime, thinly sliced

Preheat the broiler.

Arrange fillets on a baking sheet or in a baking dish and sprinkle them with pepper. Then, using a pastry brush, brush them with the oil. Brush the mustard evenly over the fish.

Put fillets into broiler, about 3 inches from heat source. Broil for about 2 minutes, or until golden brown. Do not overcook. Place on individual dishes sprinkled with chives and lay lime slices on top of the fish.

Broiled Swordfish with Sautéed Sweet Onions

SERVES 4

Marilu: This Spanish swordfish is a great combination of flavors.

Tasters' comments: The "sweet onion works so well with the swordfish." "It's lovely with the tomato."

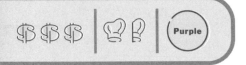

3 tablespoons extra-virgin olive oil

5 cups thinly sliced onions

Salt

½ cup water

Freshly ground pepper

1 teaspoon finely chopped fresh rosemary

1 can (14.5 ounces) chopped tomatoes, or 1½ cups peeled and chopped vine-ripened tomatoes

1 tablespoon Sucanat

1½ tablespoons finely chopped fresh flat-leaf parsley

4 swordfish steaks, about 7 ounces each, at least 1 inch thick

Lemon wedges

Heat 2 tablespoons of the olive oil in a large sauté pan over medium heat until hot. Add the onions and a little salt so the onions release their liquid. Reduce heat to medium-low and sauté until onions stop releasing liquid and pan is nearly dry again, about 4 minutes. Do not allow the onions to brown. Add the water, cover, and cook, stirring occasionally, until the onions are very soft, about 10 minutes.

Uncover, season with pepper, add the rosemary, and increase heat to medium-high. Sauté until the onions are very lightly browned, about 10 minutes. Remove half of the onions to a plate and set aside.

Add the tomatoes and their juice to the onions remaining in the pan. Bring to a boil over high heat, season with salt and pepper, lower the heat, and simmer until thick, about 4 minutes. Add the Sucanat. Remove from heat and let cool for a bit. Stir in 1 tablespoon of the parsley. (The recipe may be completed up to this point a day ahead. Cover and refrigerate the reserved onions and sauce separately.)

Preheat oven to 450 degrees. Turn on the broiler, if a separate unit. Heat the remaining olive oil in a large, ovenproof sauté pan over medium-high heat until hot. Season the fish steaks with salt and pepper and place in pan. Place in oven. Broil until the fish is browned on the underside, about 1½ minutes. Turn and top evenly with the reserved onions.

To serve, reheat the sauce, if necessary. It should be warm, not blistering hot. Pour the sauce onto a serving platter or divide among 4 plates. Top with the fish, dust with the remaining ½ tablespoon parsley, and serve immediately with lemon wedges.

Mussels Sautéed with Tomato

SERVES 4 AS FIRST COURSE, 2 AS MAIN COURSE

Marilu: *A mussel lover's dream.*

Tasters' comments: *"Great starter." "This looks impressive but it's so easy to make."*

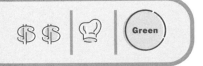

2 tablespoons extra-virgin olive oil

1½ tablespoons sliced garlic

1½ pounds mussels, scrubbed and debearded

1 cup vermouth

Salt and freshly ground pepper

3 large yellow tomatoes, peeled and cut into chunks about the same size as the mussels

1 tablespoon finely chopped fresh purple or green basil

1½ teaspoons finely chopped fresh tarragon

1½ teaspoons finely chopped fresh flat-leaf parsley

2 tablespoons soy margarine

Heat the olive oil in a large sauté pan over medium-high heat until hot. Add the garlic and sauté briefly until light brown. Add the mussels and vermouth and season with salt and pepper. Stir, then cover and cook until the mussels begin to open, about 2 minutes. As they open, transfer them with a slotted spoon to a plate. Discard any that do not open.

Cook the juices over medium-high heat until reduced by about half. Add the tomatoes and cook quickly just until they begin to color the juice, about 30 seconds. Do not overcook or they will melt into the sauce. Add the herbs and the soy margarine. When the margarine has melted, return the mussels to the pan with any juices accumulated on the plate. Stir and toss just to reheat. Serve immediately.

Steamed California Mussels
a tavola

a tavola: These mussels are prepared in the style of Liguria, Italy, where the mountains meet the sea.

Marilu: You'll want every drop of the remaining sauce. Make sure you have a side of beans so you can lap up the juice with a piece of bread and still food combine.

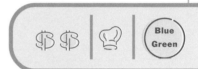

¼ cup extra-virgin olive oil
4 large cloves garlic, crushed
3 pounds California mussels
2 cups white wine (pinot grigio suggested)

4 peeled, seeded, and diced ripe plum tomatoes
1 bunch chopped Italian parsley leaves

Slowly heat olive oil with garlic until golden brown. In a very hot, heavy pot with a tight-fitting lid, add garlic oil, mussels, wine, tomatoes, and half of the parsley. Shake briefly to mix and cook approximately 2 minutes until mussels are just opened. Discard any that don't open.

Arrange open mussels on a warm serving platter. Slightly reduce liquid and pour over the top of the mussels. Add remaining parsley and serve with a crusty bread.

Sea Bass in Molasses Sauce

SERVES 4

Marilu: This is one of my favorite fish. It has such a succulent flavor.

Tasters' comments: "What a flaky and flavorful moist fish."

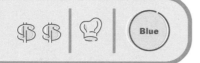

Fish

Two 1-inch-thick fillets Chilean sea bass, skinned

1 teaspoon ground cumin

⅛ teaspoon salt

⅛ teaspoon pepper

¼ teaspoon olive oil

Sauce

1 cup vegetable broth

2 tablespoons molasses

¼ cup fresh lime juice

1 teaspoon kuzu or cornstarch

Preheat oven to 500 degrees.

Pat fillets dry and sprinkle with cumin and salt and pepper to taste on both sides. Heat oil in a well-seasoned 10-inch cast-iron skillet over high heat until hot but not smoking, then sear fillets until browned on one side, about 5 minutes. Turn fillets over and put skillet in oven. Roast fillets in upper third of oven until just cooked through, 6 to 8 minutes.

Whisk together broth, molasses, juice, and kuzu in a small skillet and simmer, whisking, until slightly thickened, 4 to 5 minutes. Halve each fillet crosswise. Spoon sauce over and around fish and serve.

Halibut with Checca over Couscous

Marilu: This pretty presentation is a very light dish. If you served a bean dish for an appetizer, you would have a perfect food combination. Makes a great summer lunch.

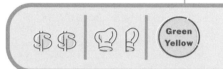

2 tomatoes, chopped

2 cloves garlic, chopped

4 basil leaves, chopped

1 teaspoon olive oil

Salt and pepper to taste

4 halibut fillets

1 cup couscous

Put tomatoes, garlic, and basil in a small bowl with ½ teaspoon olive oil, salt, and pepper, and let marinate, 10 to 15 minutes.

Make the couscous according to the package directions.

Rub halibut fillets with remaining ½ teaspoon olive oil and salt and pepper. Grill four minutes a side on very hot grill.

Spoon ½ cup couscous on each plate. Place halibut fillet on top and spoon tomato mixture over fish.

Shrimp, Saffron, and Vegetable Risotto

SERVES 6

Marilu: It's so colorful. Serve with a bean first course and you have food-combining greatness.

Tasters' comments: "This is definitely a saffron lover's delight." A "great dinner-party dish."

   Green Yellow

1 small yellow onion, chopped
1 tablespoon soy margarine
1 tablespoon olive oil
1½ cups arborio rice
Salt and pepper to taste
6 to 8 cups vegetable stock

18 to 24 medium shrimp, peeled and deveined
1 cup broccoli florets
6 to 8 basil leaves
1 teaspoon saffron

Sauté onion in soy margarine and olive oil until translucent. Add arborio rice. Stir until coated. Season with salt and pepper. Start adding vegetable stock 1 cup at a time, stirring constantly.

In a separate pan over high heat, cook shrimp in a little olive oil for about 5 minutes or until pink on outside. Set aside.

Add broccoli and basil to risotto, allowing to cook until tender. Continue to add stock 1 cup at a time, stirring constantly. Add saffron and salt and pepper. Cook until al dente, about 30 minutes. Stir in the cooked shrimp.

Note: You may substitute asparagus or peas for broccoli.

Swordfish with Lentils

SERVES 4

Marilu: This rich-tasting and simple-to-prepare dish is great to serve when you want to impress a guest.

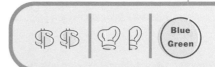

4 swordfish fillets, about 6 ounces each

Salt and pepper

1 tablespoon plus 1 teaspoon extra-virgin olive oil

1 medium shallot, thinly sliced

1 garlic clove, chopped

2 plum tomatoes, seeded and chopped

One 15-ounce can lentils

1 teaspoon vermouth

Season the fish steaks on both sides with salt and pepper. Set aside.

In a medium sauté pan, heat 1 tablespoon olive oil. Add the shallot and garlic and sauté until tender. Add the tomatoes, lentils, and vermouth and sauté for an additional 5 to 10 minutes.

In a heavy, ovenproof sauté pan over medium-high heat, heat 1 teaspoon olive oil until hot. Add the fish and sear for about 2 minutes on each side. For each serving, place a piece of fish in the center of a scoop of lentil mixture.

Poached Salmon with Sherry-Shallot Mayonnaise and Black Beans

Bread & Butter Catering

SERVES 4

Marilu: You'll impress your friends with this delicious entrée that's easy to make.

Tasters' comments: "The salmon, beans, and mayo complement each other perfectly."

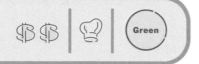

Mayonnaise

1 medium shallot, chopped

1 small garlic clove, chopped

⅓ cup dry sherry

**4 tablespoons canned black beans,
rinsed and drained, half of them
chopped**

1 teaspoon soy sauce

1½ cups Nayonaise

Salmon

Four 6-ounce skinless salmon fillets

1½ cups white wine

1 bay leaf

3 sprigs fresh dill

1 teaspoon whole black peppercorns

Place all mayonnaise ingredients except Nayonaise in small heavy-bottomed saucepan and cook until reduced by half. Allow to cool. Place salmon fillets, white wine, bay leaf, dill, and peppercorns in baking dish and add enough water to cover. Cover dish. Poach in a 350-degree oven for 10 to 15 minutes until just cooked through. Now, fold cooled mayonnaise mixture into the Nayonaise (or substitute any prepared vegetarian mayonnaise). Serve alongside the fish.

Simple Swordfish

Tasters' comments: *"Rich and simple." "I'm a sucker for a good firm piece of swordfish."*

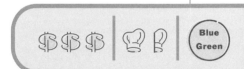

1¼ tablespoons soy sauce

¼ teaspoon minced garlic

¼ teaspoon grated lemon peel

1 tablespoon lemon juice

½ teaspoon Dijon mustard

2 tablespoons olive oil

Four 8-ounce swordfish fillets

1 pound vegetables of your choice,
   broiled or grilled

Blend first six ingredients together in a blender or food processor until emulsified. Reserve half in a bowl. Pour remaining liquid into baking pan. Add fish and marinate for 15 to 20 minutes. Broil or grill swordfish using reserved liquid to baste. Serve with vegetables.

Halibut with Jicama and Beans

Tasters' comments: "A summer's night fish dish or great for when you want something light." "This is a great lunch or dinner."

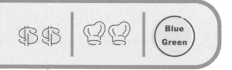

3 large vine-ripened tomatoes	1½ cups chopped jicama
¾ cup extra-virgin olive oil	2 tablespoons white wine vinegar
1 teaspoon minced garlic	1 tablespoon finely chopped fresh
1 tablespoon freshly squeezed lemon juice	tarragon
	½ cup soy bacon bits
Salt and freshly ground pepper	4 halibut fillets, about 5 ounces
1 cup shelled lima beans, fava beans, or other fresh shelling beans	each

Core the tomatoes, cut into pieces, and place in a blender. Blend until pureed. Strain through a sieve into a bowl. You should have about 1½ cups puree.

Heat 1 tablespoon olive oil in a nonreactive medium saucepan until hot. Add the garlic and sauté briefly until light brown. Add the tomato puree and bring to a boil. Simmer gently about 5 minutes. Strain through a fine-mesh sieve into a bowl. Discard the solids.

Rinse out the saucepan, return the tomato juice to the pan, and bring to a boil. Simmer and strain twice more until the tomato juice is as thick as heavy cream, about 15 minutes total cooking time. Be sure to lower the heat as the mixture thickens to prevent scorching. You should have about ¼ cup of very smooth tomato juice. Add the lemon juice and taste for salt and pepper.

Pour 1 tablespoon olive oil into a small, clean glass bottle with a stopper and swirl to coat the inside. Strain the tomato juice into the bottle. Let it cool to room temperature. Add 2 tablespoons of the olive oil. Do not shake or mix!

Cook beans in water just until tender, about 3 minutes. Drain. If using favas, peel them. Toss with fresh jicama in a bowl.

In a clean jar with a lid, shake together the vinegar, tarragon, 3 tablespoons of the soy bacon bits, and 6 tablespoons olive oil. Pour enough of the dressing onto the jicama and beans to coat, toss well, and taste for seasoning. Adjust with salt, pepper, and more dressing as necessary. Set aside to marinate for about 15 minutes.

Season the fish on both sides with salt and pepper. Heat the remaining 2 tablespoons olive oil in a large sauté pan over medium-high heat until hot. Add the fish and cook until brown on the first side, about 3 minutes. Turn and continue to cook until opaque throughout, about 3 minutes longer. Remove from the pan and keep warm.

When ready to serve, pile the bean mixture on a platter or divide among 4 large plates. Arrange the fish on top of the salad. Shake the tomato vinaigrette bottle gently. You do not want the mixture to emulsify, but to have separate droplets suspended within the oil. Spoon or shake about 1 tablespoon of the "broken" tomato vinaigrette on each piece of halibut and then drizzle or shake more tomato vinaigrette around the edges of the platter or plates. Garnish with the remaining soy bacon bits.

Bow-Tie Pasta with Salmon and White Beans

MaryAnn Hennings

SERVES 6 TO 8

Marilu: This is one of the team's favorites.

Tasters' comments: "This has a great combo of flavors." "The dill with the salmon mixes so well." "Sooo good."

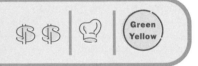

1 pound farfalle (bow-tie pasta)

2 cloves garlic

2 tablespoons Dijon mustard

¼ cup red wine vinegar

¼ cup fresh lemon juice

6 tablespoons olive oil

2 tablespoons soy sour cream

1 pound smoked salmon, cut in strips

One 15-ounce can white beans

⅓ cup chopped fresh parsley

⅓ cup chopped fresh dill

2 to 4 tablespoons capers

1 small red onion, chopped

Coarsely ground black pepper

½ cup soy Parmesan

Bring a large pot of water to boil. Add pasta and cook until tender. Drain immediately. Transfer pasta to a large mixing bowl.

While the pasta is cooking, make the dressing. Place garlic in a blender or in a food processor fitted with a steel blade; pulse until chunky. Add mustard, vinegar, and lemon juice, and process until combined. Gradually add olive oil and soy sour cream.

Pour dressing over pasta. Add salmon, beans, parsley, dill, capers, and red onion. Mix together.

Add pepper to taste. Top with soy Parmesean.

Fettuccine with White Clam Sauce

SERVES 4

Tasters' comments: *"When you're in the mood for an Italian night, serve this with a nice crusty bread and light bean salad." "This is the kind of pasta you eat with a spoon and fork."*

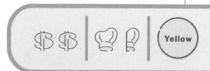

2 dozen medium to large clams

1 tablespoon chopped shallots

½ cup olive oil

1 teaspoon chopped garlic

2 tablespoons chopped parsley

¼ teaspoon dried red hot peppers

¼ cup white wine or vermouth

1 tablespoon soy margarine

2 tablespoons grated soy Parmesan

Salt to taste

1 pound fettuccine

Put clams in large bowl of cold water, let stand for 5 minutes. Drain, refill the bowl with clean water. Scrub the clams vigorously with a coarse stiff brush. Rinse and repeat process until clams are clean.

Put the shallots in a small saucepan with the olive oil, and sauté over medium-high heat until translucent. Add the garlic and sauté until lightly colored. Add the parsley and hot pepper, stir for just about 30 seconds, and add the wine or vermouth. Allow the wine to boil until it's reduced by half.

Rinse the clams in their own juices and chop them into small pieces. Filter the clam juice through a sieve lined with paper towels. You should have about ⅔ cup of liquid.

Add the clams to the saucepan. Turn them quickly in the hot sauce and turn the heat off. Add the soy margarine and the soy Parmesan, mixing thoroughly. Add salt if necessary. Make the fettuccine according to the directions on the box.

When the fettuccine is ready, drain it, pour the clam sauce over the top, and serve.

Linguine with Red Clam Sauce

Joe Rowley

SERVES 4 TO 6

Marilu: My son Joey had 3 helpings. Everybody thought it was fantastic. It became Lizzy's favorite, and she doesn't like clams.

Tasters' comments: "A culinary delight."

3 cans whole baby clams

One and a half 28-ounce cans peeled plum tomatoes

1 finely chopped medium-size red onion

1 cup finely chopped fresh flat-leaf parsley

6 large cloves garlic, chopped

¼ cup extra-virgin olive oil

1 teaspoon dried chili flakes

Coarse salt

⅓ cup dry white wine

1 tablespoon dried oregano

Freshly ground black pepper

1 pound fettuccine or linguine

One 15-ounce can black beans

Strain the water from the clams into a bowl. Do this first so that any sediment from the clams will settle to the bottom, allowing you to use some of the clam juice in the sauce.

Put a pot of salted water on the stove to boil.

Coarsely chop the tomatoes; reserve in their liquid. Prepare the red onion and parsley; and peel, smash, and chop the garlic. Although you're now ready to cook, listen up.

The order in which the ingredients are cooked is important. If you just throw it all together, the clams will have the taste and texture of a rubber eraser.

Over medium to high heat, add the olive oil and chili flakes to the pan and cook for about a minute. The chilies will soften and give up some of their oil. Add the chopped onion along with some coarse salt and sauté until translucent and soft—the sign that the onion has given up its sugar. Add the garlic and cook for 1 to 2 minutes. Sauté it longer and you risk burning it. If you do, the sauce will be bitter.

Pour the white wine in the pan and allow it to boil down by half.

Now add the chopped tomatoes with their liquid, along with the oregano and about half of the parsley. Season the mixture with about 10 grinds of black pepper from your pepper mill. Sauté it all (stirring frequently) until most of the water has cooked off and the flesh of the tomatoes has softened and broken down, leaving a thick pasty sauce. It should take 20 to 25 minutes.

Drop the fettuccine or linguine into the boiling water in your pasta pot before the sauce is done. That way the noodles and sauce should be finished cooking at about the same time—the pasta should take 10 to 13 minutes to cook al dente. You'll feel like a genius of culinary timing.

Stir black beans into the sauce and cook for 1 to 2 minutes. Then stir the drained clams into the sauce, and add small amounts of the clam juice until the sauce has a "thick soup" consistency—the thickness of, say, split pea or other pureed soup. The point here is to have a sauce that coats the pasta well, but doesn't lose its richness because there's too much water.

Cook the sauce for a final 2 or 3 minutes, making sure the clams and the sauce are heated through. Take a taste and adjust the seasoning. Don't cook it too long, though. The clams will get tough and rubbery.

Toss the noodles and sauce together, garnish with the remaining chopped parsley, serve, and acknowledge the applause.

Upside-Down Garlic Chicken

Elizabeth Carney   SERVES 4

Tasters' comments: *"Wow, this is so juicy." "I love the sweet garlic flavor."*

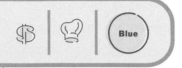

1 whole free-range chicken
1 garlic bulb
Cinnamon

Preheat oven to 350 degrees. Wash and remove insides of chicken. Cut off the end of the garlic bulb on both sides so that cloves are exposed. Place bulb inside chicken cavity.

Sprinkle the chicken with cinnamon on the inside, generously. Sprinkle cinnamon on outside of chicken as well. Place in baking pan, upside down (this will keep the breasts moist). Bake 18 to 20 minutes per pound, basting occasionally.

Roasted Chicken with Garlic and Rosemary

Beth Heffner

SERVES 4

Tasters' comments: *This "moist and succulent" dish "falls off the bone."*

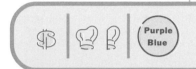

2 tablespoons soy margarine

2 tablespoons olive oil

2 garlic cloves

1 free-range chicken, about
2½ pounds, cut into quarters

Small sprig fresh rosemary

Salt and freshly ground pepper

½ cup vermouth

Heat the soy margarine and oil in a large sauté pan over medium heat. When the margarine foams, add the garlic and the chicken quarters, skin side down. When the chicken is well browned on one side, turn the pieces over and add the rosemary.

When the chicken is cooked well on both sides, add a large pinch of salt and pepper and the vermouth. Allow the vermouth to bubble for about 3 minutes, then lower the heat to a simmer and cover the pan. Cook it for about 30 to 35 minutes. Turn the chicken a couple of times while cooking. Transfer the chicken to a warm serving plate. Remove the garlic from the pan. Tilt the pan and, with a spoon, remove and discard all but 2 tablespoons of fat. Return the pan to high heat, add 2 to 3 tablespoons of water, and scrape up the cooking juices. Pour these over the chicken and serve.

Chicken with Tarragon

Joe Rowley

Marilu: My boys eat chicken (as long as it's free-range) and they loved this dish. The chicken looked so juicy.

Tasters' comments: "My God, this is so incredibly flavorful." "A meat-lover's chicken for sure."

Blue Green

2 whole free-range chicken breasts (4 fillets)
Salt and freshly ground black pepper
⅓ cup olive or sunflower oil
2 tablespoons soy margarine
½ cup chopped yellow onion

1 clove garlic, chopped
1 tablespoon chopped fresh tarragon
1 tablespoon finely chopped flat-leaf parsley
⅔ cup dry white wine
1 cup chicken stock

Take the chicken breasts from the refrigerator about 30 minutes before you begin so they can come to room temperature. Fillet the breasts, rinse the fillets with cold water, and pat dry with paper towels. Sprinkle the breasts all over with salt and freshly ground black pepper.

Heat the oil and 1 tablespoon of soy margarine in a sauté pan and sauté the breasts over medium-high heat, turning occasionally, until cooked through, about 15 to 20 minutes.

When the chicken is done, put on a plate and set in a warm oven. Pour all of the oil and chicken fat out of the sauté pan. The bottom of the pan should have brown, caramelized drippings stuck to it. That's just what you want.

Return the pan to medium-high heat, melt 1 tablespoon of soy margarine, and sauté the onion until it's translucent and soft. Add the garlic and cook for 1 to 2 minutes, stirring constantly to keep it from burning. Stir the tarragon and parsley in for another 1 to 2 minutes, allowing the flavors to mix together.

Now add the white wine to deglaze the pan. Keep stirring and scraping with a wooden spatula to remove all of that wonderful caramelized stuff from the bottom of the pan. Let the mixture boil until its volume is reduced by half, then pour in the chicken stock.

Bring the sauce back to a boil, then turn the heat down to medium low. Slice the chicken into strips and add them to the sauce. Continue cooking for 4 to 5 minutes.

Arrange the chicken strips on a platter. Pour the extra sauce over them and garnish with a light sprinkle of parsley.

Soy Entrées

EZ Sloppy Joes

Marilu: The whole family will love it.

Tasters' comments: "This is so close to the real thing." "You should try this with the kids." "Quick and easy."

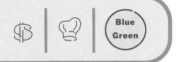

1 bag ground Boca Burger

1 package sloppy joe mix from health food store

One 15-ounce can pizza/pasta sauce

Mix all ingredients together. Add water if necessary. Simmer 7 to 10 minutes. Serve hot.

Eggless Salad

Julie Pearce

Julie: *Many ethnic cookbooks seem to follow the food-combining principles—I have seen several Indian and Thai cookbooks that look really wonderful (although I haven't actually purchased any yet). This is a really easy recipe I like for sandwiches (when served on bread, it makes a complete protein). You may need to adjust the ingredients to your taste.*

Marilu: *I really liked this flavor, and the dish keeps well for a few days.*

Tasters' comments: *"What a great protein dish for lunch." "This makes a fantastic sandwich filler!"*

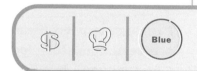

1 pound drained extra-firm tofu
Nayonaise to taste (about ¼ to ½
   cup)
1 to 2 tablespoons prepared organic
   mustard
1 teaspoon cumin

1 teaspoon garlic powder
1 teaspoon onion powder
Salt and pepper to taste
1 medium carrot, chopped
Chopped scallions to taste (optional)

Thoroughly drain tofu. Mash with potato masher or fork, add Nayonaise, mustard, spices, and chopped vegetables, if desired. Refrigerate for at least 1 hour to allow flavors to mix. Serve on whole-grain bread.

Tofu Tacos

SERVES 4

Marilu: The flavor is great and it's an interesting change from regular tacos.

Tasters' comments: "You need more of an adult palate for this." "These are great if you like the firmness of tofu."

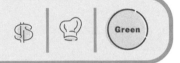

1 package taco mix (**Bearritos brand is best**) from health food store

1 package extra-firm tofu, diced or cut into strips

8 corn tortillas or taco shells

1 cup chopped tomatoes

1 cup chopped onions

1 cup chopped avocado

1 cup chopped lettuce

Hot sauce

Optional: any other fillings you choose

Prepare the taco mix according to package instructions. Add the tofu. Have fun assembling the tacos.

Note: These can also be made using ground Boca Burger instead of tofu, which would make it a fun food to cook with the kids and good, very easy party food.

Santa Fe Wrap

Marilu: *This clean tasting, Tex-Mex influenced flavor is hearty and full of gusto.*

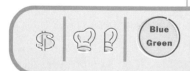

4 tablespoons fresh lime juice

1 tablespoon vegetable oil

8 ounces firm tofu, drained, patted dry, crumbled

¼ cup chopped red onion

⅓ cup chopped fresh cilantro

1 garlic clove, minced

Salt and pepper

Four 7- to 8-inch diameter flour tortillas

2 cups thinly sliced lettuce leaves

1 cup spicy tomato salsa

Whisk 3 tablespoons lime juice and oil in a medium bowl. Add tofu, onion, cilantro, and garlic and toss to blend. Season to taste with salt and pepper. Let marinate 20 minutes.

Preheat oven to 350 degrees. Wrap tortillas in foil. Place in oven until heated through, about 10 minutes.

Meanwhile, toss lettuce with 1 tablespoon lime juice in small bowl.

Place 1 tortilla on each of 4 plates. Place layer of lettuce down center of each tortilla. Top with tofu mixture, dividing equally. Spoon 1½ tablespoons salsa over each. Roll up tortillas. Serve, passing remaining salsa separately.

Coconut Curried Chowder

Suzanne "Suzall" Palumbo   SERVES 6

Suzanne: *The longer this sits, the more curry it takes on (i.e., it's better the next day). But I thought it kicked butt 1 hour later. I drained the tofu like the recipe said. I checked about coconut milk; the brand I used had no dairy. (Some manufacturers boil coconut in dairy milk, don't buy these.) I love curry, so you might want to adjust. Go for the gusto!*

Marilu: *A curry lover's dream.*

2 teaspoons vegetable oil

⅔ cup chopped onion

3 chopped green onions, white and green parts separated

1 cup peeled, diced sweet potato

⅓ cup diced sweet red pepper

3 teaspoons grated peeled fresh ginger

2 cloves chopped garlic

3 cups fat-free chicken or vegetable broth

One 14-ounce can light coconut milk

½ cup frozen or fresh corn kernels

2½ teaspoons curry powder

½ teaspoon grated lemon zest

⅛ teaspoon cayenne (optional)

¼ teaspoon salt

10 ounces extra-firm tofu, drained and preferably pressed, cut into bite-size chunks

2 tablespoons chopped fresh cilantro leaves (optional)

In large pot, heat oil over medium low. Add onion and white part of green onions. Sauté 2 minutes. Add sweet potato, red pepper, 2 teaspoons of the ginger, and garlic. Sauté 3 minutes. Stir in broth and heat until boiling. Reduce heat to low, cover, and simmer 10 to 15 minutes or until sweet potato is tender.

Add coconut milk, corn, curry, lemon zest, cayenne, salt, and remaining ginger and green onion. Gently stir tofu into soup mixture. Remove from heat and let stand for at least 30 minutes to allow tofu to absorb seasonings. Just before serving, reheat soup over low heat (do not boil). Stir in cilantro, if desired, and serve.

PRESSING AND DRAINING TOFU

1. Cut block of tofu in half horizontally to make two slabs.
2. Cover a cutting board with aluminum foil and prop it up slightly so it slants and drains into the sink. Place tofu slabs on the board.
3. Cover tofu with a second layer of foil; place a baking sheet on top to cover. Weight it with heavy cans or books and let stand at least 20 minutes.

Hunter's Tofu

Pat Erickson

Pat: *This recipe was originally an Adirondack Mountain meat recipe called "Hunter's Chicken." I have modified it using tofu. It still has the same satisfying taste and is a great winter "got to get warm" dish. It will make you smile!*

Marilu: *I love this dish. The flavors sit so well on your palate you can't stop eating it.*

Tasters' Comments: *"Interesting blend of flavors." "Cozy food."*

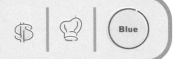

1 package extra-firm tofu
Whole-wheat flour for dredging
Olive oil for frying
Pinch of fresh chopped or powdered
    garlic
1 cup vegetable bouillon

3 small vine-ripened tomatoes,
    squashed
2 tablespoons fresh chopped parsley
    plus more for garnish
¼ cup diced shallots
¼ cup white zinfandel

To achieve the right consistency in this dish you must first freeze the tofu. After thawing it, press out all the water gently with paper towels. This makes the tofu easier to slice.

Slice the tofu into 1-inch sections. Gently roll these sections in whole wheat flour so they are just lightly dusted. Quickly brown each section in olive oil with a pinch of garlic added. Remove the sections and allow them to drain on a towel.

In another large frying pan, place tofu, vegetable bouillon, tomatoes, parsley, shallots, and zinfandel. Simmer for 1 hour. Top with parsley leaves.

Comfort Pasta

Renee Scott

SERVES 4 TO 6

Renee: I am new to this site, but I've been with the program for over a year. This is my favorite "comfort food" recipe. My little cousins and my boyfriend love it—even after I tell them it's soy cheese!

Marilu: Great with a video on a rainy night.

Tasters' comments: "It's so easy and the kids love it." "Tastes like the real thing."

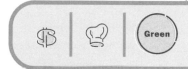

1 box wheatless elbow pasta
1 package Mori-Nu firm tofu
1 brick (12 ounces) grated mild cheddar soy cheese (I like Soya Kaas)

1 pat soy butter (optional)
¼ cup plain soy milk

Cook the pasta according to package directions. In a blender or food processor, blend the tofu until it is smooth and without lumps. Transfer the tofu to a saucepan, and stir in the cheese over medium heat. Continue to stir, making sure not to let the sauce boil. Add the pat of soy butter to the pasta (optional) before pouring the sauce mixture on top. Add the soy milk as needed as you stir the pasta and sauce together. And there you have the ultimate dairy-free comfort food!

Note: Sometimes I add sautéed broccoli and diced onions to the mix—it's a good way to get my little cousins to eat their vegetables!

Enchiladas with Sautéed Peppers

SERVES 6

Marilu: *This is a great dish for a festive party. Toss in the oven and forget about it for 15 minutes. It's great and hearty.*

1 tablespoon olive oil

1 chopped red onion

1 green bell pepper, sliced in strips

1 red bell pepper, sliced in strips

1 teaspoon chili powder

2 cans enchilada sauce

12 corn tortillas

3 cups grated soy or rice cheese (rice cheese melts and tastes better)

2 cups chopped cilantro

1 cup chopped green onions

1 cup sliced black olives

Preheat oven to 375 degrees. Heat olive oil in skillet. Add red onion. Sauté at medium heat for 2 minutes. Add bell peppers. Turn heat to medium-low. Gradually add chili powder to taste. Sauté until peppers are tender, then set aside. In casserole dish, pour ½ cup enchilada sauce, so dish is coated with a thin layer. Pour the rest of the sauce in a large bowl. Take one tortilla and saturate in sauce, then lay in casserole dish. In center of tortilla, sprinkle cheese, cilantro, green onions, sautéed onions and peppers, and olives.

Fold tortilla and lay folded edge facedown on casserole dish. Repeat until casserole dish is filled. Pour a small amount of sauce over whole dish. Generously sprinkle the rest of the cheese over the folded tortillas. Dress the dish with olives, green onions, and cilantro and cook for 15 to 20 minutes until cheese is thoroughly melted and enchilada sauce bubbles. Let cool a few minutes and serve.

Manicotti

Marilu: *What a fantastic manicotti, and you don't miss the ricotta. I love being able to redo old favorites for my new way of life.*

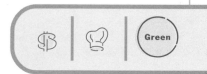

1 head garlic

2 pounds tofu

2 teaspoons salt

¾ cup plus 2 tablespoons olive oil

1 finely chopped large onion

½ cup finely chopped fresh parsley

1 package manicotti noodles

6 cups Italian-style tomato sauce

Cut off top of garlic so that all cloves are exposed. Drizzle with olive oil. Place on baking sheet and bake at 350 degrees for 20 minutes. Remove 5 cloves (save the rest for another use) and blend them with tofu, salt, and ¾ cup of olive oil in a blender until smooth and creamy.

Bring a pot of salted water to a boil. In a small skillet, sauté together 2 tablespoons of olive oil and the onion. Fold sautéed onions into tofu mixture along with the parsley.

Drop manicotti noodles into boiling water and boil for about 10 minutes or until noodles are almost al dente. Drain and rinse.

Pour 2 cups of tomato sauce on the bottom of a 9 x 13-inch pan. Fill each cooked noodle with ⅓ to ½ cup of filling. Line up the filled noodles in the pan and cover with the rest of the sauce. Bake in a 350-degree oven for about 30 minutes and serve.

Shepherd's Pie

Chicago Diner

MAKES 1 PIE

Marilu: *This warm and cozy meal is a redo of the old-time favorite. It is very hearty, with a savory flavor.*

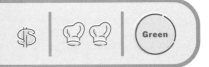

1 cup lentils

2 cups water

1 bay leaf

1 package tempeh

1 tablespoon tamari or soy sauce

1 tablespoon Bragg Liquid Aminos

1 tablespoon oil

1 coarsely chopped medium onion

1 coarsely chopped carrot

2 coarsely chopped stalks celery

1 cup coarsely chopped mushrooms

1 teaspoon sage

1 teaspoon thyme

1 teaspoon marjoram

½ teaspoon salt

⅛ teaspoon pepper

2 pounds peeled potatoes

2 tablespoons soy margarine

¼ teaspoon nutmeg

¼ cup soy milk

Sort and wash lentils. Boil the water, add the bay leaf and lentils, cover, and cook until lentils are soft, approximately 25 minutes.

Preheat oven to 350 degrees. Cube and toss the tempeh with tamari and Bragg's. Place cubes on a cookie sheet and bake for 15 minutes. Leave oven on.

In a sauté pan over medium-high heat, add oil and sauté onion, carrot, celery, mushrooms, sage, thyme, marjoram, salt, and pepper. Cook until soft, approximately 8 to 10 minutes. Add cooked lentils and tempeh; mix well and pour into casserole pan. Set aside and prepare potato mixture.

Place peeled potatoes in pot of water. Boil until soft when tested with a fork. Drain potatoes and return to pot. Add margarine, nutmeg, and salt and pepper to taste. Mash until soft, adding soy milk to achieve desired consistency. Cover casserole with potato mixture and bake, uncovered, for 45 minutes.

Spicy Chili over Polenta à la Joy

Joy Leinoff

Marilu: *This spicy chili was a hit with everyone.*

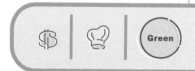

2 to 3 tablespoons olive oil

2 large onions, cut into ½-inch dice

1 red pepper, cut into ½-inch chunks

1 yellow pepper, cut into ½-inch chunks

2 zucchini, cut into ½-inch chunks

4 to 6 cloves garlic, minced

2 tablespoons good-quality chili powder

One 32-ounce can Italian tomatoes in their juice, cut into ½-inch dice

1 pound plum tomatoes, cut into ½-inch dice

1 tablespoon ground cumin

1 tablespoon dried basil

1 tablespoon dried oregano

1 teaspoon fennel seeds

Kosher salt and freshly ground pepper

1 can red beans, drained (Goya is best)

2 quarts water

2 cups dairy-free polenta

Chopped fresh scallions to taste

Grated Monterey Jack soy cheese to taste

Heat 2 tablespoons olive oil in large Dutch oven. Add onions and peppers and sauté until translucent, about 8 minutes. Add zucchini and continue sautéing another 3 to 4 minutes or so. Add garlic, chili powder, canned tomatoes, fresh tomatoes, cumin, basil, oregano, fennel seeds, and salt and pepper to taste. Cook, stirring often, for 20 minutes. Add red beans. Adjust the seasonings to taste, and cook for an additional 10 minutes or so. Cover and refrigerate overnight.

Bring 2 quarts of water to a boil. Add 1 tablespoon kosher salt. Stir in polenta, whisking with wire whisk the whole time, until polenta is smooth.

First, fill bowl with polenta, then spoon chili over to cover. Top with fresh scallion and grated Monterey Jack soy cheese. Enjoy.

Super Bowl Chili

MaryAnn Hennings

MAKES APPROXIMATELY 8 CUPS

Tasters' comments: *"This is a great meat lover's dish." "It tastes so good, it seems bad for you, but it's not!"*

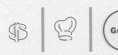

1 teaspoon olive oil

1 chopped medium Spanish onion

4 cloves garlic, chopped or pressed

1 pound soy meat (Gimme Lean or
    ground Boca Burger)

1 to 3 tablespoons chili powder

2 tablespoons dried oregano

1 teaspoon ground cumin

1 teaspoon ground cinnamon

1 cup vegetable stock

One 28-ounce can crushed tomatoes

Two 16-ounce cans dark red kidney
    beans, drained and rinsed

2 tablespoons Bragg Liquid Aminos

Salt and pepper to taste

Heat the oil in a large skillet over medium-low heat. When oil is hot, add the onion and garlic and cook until golden, about 5 minutes. Add the soy meat, herbs, and spices, and cook until the soy meat is well browned. Remove any excess fat from the pan. Add the vegetable stock and simmer for about 1 hour, or until the soy meat is tender. Do not let it boil.

Add the tomatoes and beans, and cook for 20 to 30 minutes, or until the beans have softened a bit.

Add Bragg's and salt and pepper to taste, and serve with your choice of toppings (scallions, soy cheese, soy sour cream, for example).

MaryAnn's Meat Loaf

MaryAnn Hennings

SERVES 6 TO 8

Marilu: An old favorite. It actually got a "two thumbs up, baby." Also great for next-day lunches.

Tasters' comments: "It's hard to believe that it's vegetarian." It has a "great texture."

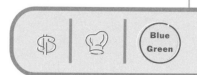

1 teaspoon olive oil

1 small Spanish onion, chopped

2 to 3 cloves garlic, finely chopped or pressed

1 teaspoon dried oregano

2 slices wheat bread

1 cup "No" Beef Broth or vegetable broth

2 large eggs, lightly beaten

2 pounds Gimme Lean (ground soy meat substitute)

¾ cup soy milk

3 tablespoons Dijon mustard

1 teaspoon black pepper

¼ to ½ teaspoon salt

¾ cup ketchup or barbecue sauce

½ cup chopped fresh parsley or cilantro

Preheat oven to 350 degrees. Lightly grease an 8 x 4-inch loaf pan.

Heat a medium-size skillet over medium heat and add the oil. When oil is hot, add the onion and cook about 3 to 5 minutes, or until golden. Reduce heat to low, add the garlic and oregano, and cook 3 minutes. Place in a large mixing bowl and set aside to cool.

In the meantime, soak the bread in the broth until moist. Squeeze excess liquid out of the bread. Add the bread to the cooled onion mixture.

Add the eggs and Gimme Lean to remaining ingredients and mix, by hand, until everything is thoroughly incorporated. Place the mixture in a loaf pan. Bake for about 1 hour and 15 minutes.

Grain and Pasta Entrées

Rich Man's Stew

Marilu: I think this recipe was the most faxed to friends and family. Everybody thinks it's great and so easy to make. Best part is, it's so low in fat.

Tasters' comments: "This is so great." "Joey wanted it in his lunch box."

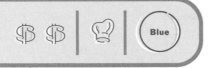

1 tablespoon olive oil

1 small red onion, diced

3 garlic cloves, minced

2 cups chopped portobello mushrooms

1 small green pepper, chopped

6 cups vegetable stock

2 plum tomatoes, chopped

1½ cups red lentils

1 bunch basil, coarsely chopped

¼ cup balsamic vinegar

Freshly ground black pepper

Heat the olive oil in large soup pot and sauté the onion, garlic, mushrooms, and green pepper (about 5 minutes).

Add vegetable stock and tomatoes to the pot and mix well. Stir in lentils and bring to a boil, then lower heat, cover, and cook over medium-low heat for 15 minutes, stirring occasionally. Add the basil and balsamic vinegar and simmer with the pot covered for another 15 minutes. Add pepper to taste and serve.

Castilian Rice

SERVES 4

Marilu: This is a dish based on Border Grill's Sea Bass Veracruz. It's a cheaper way to go and a great one-dish meal for a spicy carb night. This hot and delicious soup is great with rice. Sometimes you crave the flavor but not the fish to food combine. We substituted veggie stock for fish stock.

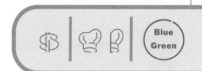

¼ cup olive oil

1 small yellow onion, thinly sliced

2 garlic cloves, minced

1 lime, cut into 8 wedges

2 jalapeños, cut into ⅛-inch discs

2 cups white wine

One 15-ounce can white beans

1 cup vegetable stock

2 tomatoes, cored, seeded, and sliced

1 bag fresh spinach

1 cup dry basmati rice, cooked according to package directions

Heat large sauté pan. Add oil and onion. Cook for 2 to 3 minutes. Add garlic, lime wedges, and jalapeños. Cook for 1 additional minute. Add white wine and let boil. Add white beans, vegetable stock, and tomatoes, and simmer for 5 minutes. Serve over raw spinach and rice.

Sierra Stew

Julie Pearce

SERVES 4 TO 6

Julie: This is more of a chili than a stew. My entire family (even the true-blue meat lovers) really enjoys it. It's very easy to make, especially when using organic canned beans, tomatoes, et cetera.

Marilu: Satisfied the toughest tasters.

Tasters' comments: "This has a hearty, Spanish flavor." "It's so easy to cook and so good."

2 tablespoons olive oil

1 large onion, thinly sliced

4 large cloves garlic, minced

1 green bell pepper, seeded and coarsely chopped

1 cup coarsely chopped green or purple cabbage

1½ cups (or more, as you desire) diced russet potatoes, unpeeled and cut in large chunks

One 16-ounce can stewed tomatoes (including liquid) or equivalent amount of fresh tomatoes

One 8-ounce can tomato sauce

1½ tablespoons chili powder (or more to taste)

¾ teaspoon ground cumin

1 large vegetarian vegetable bouillon cube

½ cup uncooked brown rice

One 15-ounce can kidney beans, rinsed and drained

Salt and pepper to taste

Toppings

Grated soy cheese or nutritional yeast flakes

Soy sour cream

Corn chips or tortilla chips

In a large Dutch oven or 8-quart pot, heat olive oil over medium-high heat. Sauté onion and garlic until onion is soft, about 3 to 5 minutes. Add bell pepper, cabbage, potatoes, tomatoes with liquid, tomato sauce, chili powder, and cumin. Continue cooking, stirring frequently, for 3 to 5 minutes. Dissolve bouillon cube in 2 cups hot or boiling water; add to mixture. Add rice, cover, and cook on low heat for approximately 90 minutes, until stew is thick and potatoes are tender. Add beans, stir, and cook, covered, for at least 30 more minutes. Season with salt and pepper, as desired. Serve topped with soy cheese, soy sour cream, and corn chips.

●   ●   ●

Variations: This stew may be made in a Crock-Pot; cook for approximately 5 hours on low heat before adding beans, cook approximately 1 hour more after adding beans. You may also use dried beans instead of canned beans; beans must be soaked overnight before adding to stew. If you use dried rather than canned beans, add beans when you add rice and vegetable broth.

Wild Mushroom Polenta

MaryAnn Hennings

SERVES 4

Tasters' comments: *"This is a very impressive dish. Not only does it look beautiful, but it tastes like it comes from a four-star restaurant."*

Blue
Green

6 tablespoons olive oil
1 cup minced shallots
3 large cloves garlic, minced
3 pounds sliced mushrooms
   (shiitake, cremini, oyster, or any
   combination)

3 teaspoons minced fresh thyme
Salt and pepper
1 box polenta mix, cooked according
   to package directions
6 tablespoons minced fresh parsley,
   for garnish

Heat the olive oil in a large skillet over moderately high heat. Add the shallots and cook, stirring, for 2 minutes, or until softened. Add the garlic and cook, stirring, 1 minute.

    Add the mushrooms, thyme, and salt and pepper to taste, and cook the mixture over moderate heat, stirring occasionally, for 5 to 7 minutes, or until the mushrooms are firm and the liquid has evaporated. Spoon the mushroom mixture over the polenta and garnish with parsley.

Chicago Diner's Oatburgers

Marilu: *This gourmet veggie burger has a unique, nutty flavor. It's one of my favorites at the Chicago Diner.*

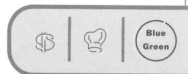

1 tablespoon soy oil or light cooking oil

1 small onion, diced

1 stalk celery, diced

2 cloves garlic, minced

Optional: chopped spinach, portobello mushrooms, or other vegetables

1½ cups water

¼ cup tamari

1 tablespoon sunflower seeds

1 tablespoon dried basil

2 teaspoons dried oregano

3 cups quick oats

½ cup whole wheat flour (can use spelt or oat flour to make wheat free)

In a 4-quart pot, heat oil and sauté onion, celery, garlic, and any other vegetables desired for 2 to 3 minutes. Add the water, tamari, sunflower seeds, basil, and oregano. Bring to a boil, then turn off. Add the oats and flour and mix well.

Let cool, then scoop out onto oiled cookie sheet to make patties. Bake at 350 degrees for 25 minutes until light brown, then flip over. Bake approximately 10 more minutes until golden.

Lentil Tacos

Ruth A. Johnson

Marilu: The kids and I loved it.

Tasters' comments: *"What an interesting change to the traditional taco." "Lots of flavor."*

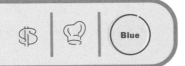

1 teaspoon olive oil

1 cup minced onions

½ cup minced celery

1 clove garlic, minced

1 cup red lentils

1 tablespoon chili powder

2 teaspoons ground cumin

1 teaspoon dried oregano

2 cups vegetable stock or broth

1 cup salsa

8 whole wheat tortillas

Toppings

Shredded greens

Chopped tomatoes

Soy cheddar cheese (optional)

In large frying pan over medium heat, add the olive oil and sauté onions, celery, and garlic for 5 minutes. Stir in lentils, chili powder, cumin, and oregano. Cook for 1 minute. Add the stock. Cover and cook for 20 minutes, or until lentils are tender. Remove the lid and cook, stirring often, until the lentils are thickened, about 10 minutes. Add salsa. Wrap the tortillas in a damp paper towel and microwave on high for 1 minute. Fill tortillas with mixture and toppings.

Curried Sweet Potato Stew

Susan Spillers

Susan: I love this recipe because it is so colorful, easy, delicious, and healthy! I became a Marilu convert after I saw you on the carousel at the Santa Monica Pier a year ago. I admired how slim, youthful, and confident you looked. I knew I wanted that! I bought your book, and even though it appeared pretty extreme at first, your program was much easier to implement than I expected. Soon, my lifelong allergies vanished, I lost ten pounds, my skin cleared up, and my cellulite faded. Thank you for sharing your healthy lifestyle with us all.

Marilu: Great Indian flavor. This light and sweet dish is a favorite with the staff. This also works really well without curry for non–curry fans.

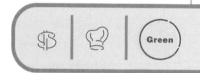

2 large sweet potatoes, peeled and
   diced
One 15-ounce can organic garbanzo
   beans, drained and rinsed
One 14.5-ounce can diced tomatoes
½ cup water
½ cup vegetable stock

10 ounces fresh spinach, coarsely
   chopped
¼ cup chopped fresh cilantro
2 green onions, chopped
2 teaspoons curry powder
½ teaspoon ground cumin
¼ teaspoon ground cinnamon

Steam sweet potatoes about 15 minutes. Meanwhile, in a large saucepan, combine garbanzo beans, tomatoes, water, and stock. Bring to a simmer over medium heat. Add spinach, cover, and cook just until wilted, about 3 minutes. Stir in sweet potatoes, cilantro, green onions, curry powder, cumin, and cinnamon. Simmer uncovered for 5 minutes.

Asparagus Shiitake Mushroom Risotto

MaryAnn Hennings   SERVES 4 AS MAIN COURSE, 8 AS SIDE DISH

Marilu: *Some fabulous vegetables with equally different textures combine to make this a winner.*

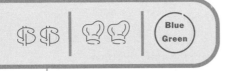

1 pound asparagus, stems and tips
   separated, stems cut in thirds
4½ cups vegetable stock
1 to 2 teaspoons olive oil
1 small white onion, finely chopped
2 cloves garlic, minced
¼ pound fresh shiitake mushrooms
   (about 8 to 10), trimmed, wiped
   clean, and thinly sliced

1½ cups arborio rice (do not substitute any other kind)
½ cup vermouth
2 tablespoons Bragg Liquid Aminos
Salt and pepper
Grated soy Parmesan (optional)

Place the asparagus stems in a large skillet with ½ cup of the stock. Bring to a boil over high heat. Reduce heat to medium, cover, and cook about 5 minutes, or until the asparagus is bright green and somewhat tender. Place in a food processor fitted with a steel blade and process until pureed. Set the puree aside. Heat the same pan over medium-low heat and add oil. When the oil is hot, add the onion, garlic, and mushrooms. Sauté until onion is golden, about 10 minutes.

Add rice and sauté 1 minute. Add vermouth and simmer until it has been completely absorbed, stirring constantly and slowly. Add stock, ½ cup at a time, until all the stock has been absorbed, continually stirring.

When you have added all the stock, add Bragg's, and when the rice is still slightly firm but tender, add the reserved asparagus puree and uncooked tips. Stir well. Add salt and pepper to taste. If desired, add soy Parmesan.

Spinach Risotto

Marilu: This very rich meal is a winner. Risotto always looks and tastes great.

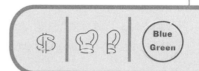

1 pound spinach	2 cups arborio rice
7 tablespoons soy margarine	½ cup vermouth
6 cups vegetable broth	½ cup soy Parmesan
1 onion, chopped	Salt and freshly ground white pepper

Wash the spinach thoroughly. Discard any yellow leaves. Drain the spinach but do not dry the leaves. In a large skillet over low heat, melt 1 tablespoon of soy margarine. Add the spinach. Cover and steam, turning and tossing occasionally to cook it evenly, or until just tender, about 5 minutes. Remove the spinach to a cutting board, and when cool enough to handle, chop it finely. Set aside.

Meanwhile, place the broth in a saucepan and bring it to a simmer. Reduce the heat to low to keep the broth hot. In a large skillet over medium heat, melt 3 tablespoons of soy margarine. Add the onion and sauté until softened, about 5 minutes. Turn the heat up to medium-high, add the rice, and continue to sauté for 1 to 2 minutes, stirring to coat well. Stir in the vermouth. Reduce the heat to medium. Allow it to evaporate and become absorbed, about 3 minutes. Now add a ladleful of hot broth, stirring well. When it is nearly all absorbed in the rice, add another ladleful of hot broth, stirring all the while.

Continue in this fashion, stirring frequently until the rice is nearly cooked. The total cooking time of the rice is 20 to 25 minutes. Mix in the spinach. After about 5 minutes, the rice will be tender but still slightly chewy. It should be creamy but not mushy. Remove it from the heat. Stir in the remaining 3 tablespoons of margarine. Add the soy cheese. Taste for salt and pepper. Serve the finished risotto piping hot, directly from the hot skillet onto plates.

Porcini Risotto

Elizabeth Carney

Marilu: This dish was inspired by Maria, a family friend from Italy. She always wowed us with her cooking.

Tasters' comments: "So my flavor." "This is a typical risotto turned upside down with the absolute mushroom madness."

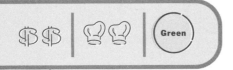

6 to 8 cups vegetable stock
3 tablespoons olive oil
½ cup finely chopped shallots
   (about 2)
1 cup arborio or carnaroli rice
½ cup white wine
1 ounce dried porcini mushrooms,
   soaked in water for 15 minutes
   and chopped

4 to 6 tablespoons soy margarine
½ cup grated soy Parmesan, plus
   extra for grating or shaving
½ cup chopped Italian parsley
Salt and freshly ground pepper

Heat stock in saucepan over medium heat; keep at a low simmer. Heat olive oil in a heavy-bottomed saucepan over medium heat. Add shallots to oil, and cook, stirring, until translucent. Add rice and cook, stirring, until rice begins to make a clicking sound like glass beads, 3 to 4 minutes.

Add wine to rice mixture. Cook, stirring, until wine is absorbed by rice.

Using a ladle, add ¾ cup hot stock to rice. Using a wooden spoon, stir rice constantly, at a moderate speed. Note: Stirring rice too vigorously will make your risotto slightly gluey; stirring too little will make it watery. Rice should be only thinly veiled in liquid during the stirring process.

When the rice mixture is just thick enough to leave a clear wake behind the spoon, add another ¾ cup stock and the porcini mushrooms.

Continue adding stock ¾ cup at a time and stirring constantly until rice is mostly translucent but still opaque in the center. Rice should be al dente but not crunchy. As rice nears doneness, watch carefully and add smaller amounts of liquid to make sure it does not overcook. The final mixture should be thick enough that grains of rice are suspended in liquid the consistency of heavy cream. It will thicken slightly when removed from heat.

Remove from heat. Stir in the soy margarine, soy Parmesan, and parsley; season with salt and pepper. Divide the mixture among 4 shallow bowls, mounding risotto in the center, and grate or shave additional Parmesan over risotto. Serve immediately.

Lentil Risotto

Marilu: *A nice change and expansion of the traditional risotto. This is a great healthy dish full of fiber and protein. I love the nice thick texture.*

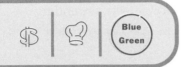

1 cup lentils

2 cups water

8 cups vegetable stock

1 tablespoon soy margarine

1 tablespoon olive oil

1 small onion, chopped

1½ cups arborio rice

Salt and pepper

¼ cup chopped Italian parsley

6 basil leaves, sliced

½ cup soy Parmesan cheese

Soak lentils overnight, unless using French lentils, which need not soak. In a medium saucepan, bring the water to a boil. Add lentils. Cook until tender, about 20 minutes. Drain and set aside.

In a saucepan over medium heat, bring stock to a simmer. In a large sauté pan over medium heat, add margarine and olive oil. Add onion and sauté until translucent. Add arborio rice and stir until coated. Season with salt and pepper. Add 4 cups of stock to the sauté pan, 1 cup at a time, until absorbed. Add lentils, parsley, and basil. Then continue to add remaining stock 1 cup at a time. Add soy cheese and season with salt and pepper to taste.

Rice Pilaf

Marilu: What a great side dish. Very flavorful.

Tasters' comments: "I would add white beans to the meal if serving a fish or protein dish as an entrée."

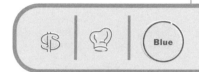

½ cup wild rice

3 shallots, chopped

1 tablespoon soy margarine

1 cup jasmine or basmati rice

Salt and pepper

¼ cup wine

2 cups boiling water

2 tablespoons chopped parsley

¼ cup toasted pine nuts

Cook wild rice according to package. Sauté shallots in soy margarine until translucent. Add jasmine or basmati rice. Stir until coated. Season with salt and pepper. Add wine. Stir until evaporated. Add boiling water. Cook 15 minutes or until water is absorbed. Let stand, covered, 5 minutes. Fluff with fork. Mix in wild rice, parsley, and toasted pine nuts. Season with salt and pepper.

Sweet Potatoes with Spinach Curry Chickpeas

Denise Barker

SERVES 4

Marilu: *I love this recipe. It has a unique flavor. The chickpeas and cilantro add something special to this dish.*

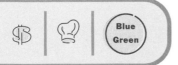

2 large sweet potatoes (about
   2 pounds), peeled and diced
One 16- to 20-ounce can chickpeas,
   rinsed and drained
One 14.5-ounce can diced tomatoes
10 to 12 ounces fresh spinach,
   stemmed and coarsely chopped
   (I have used frozen)
¼ cup chopped fresh cilantro (I find
   this a bit much, so adjust according
   to how much you like cilantro)

2 scallions, white and green parts,
   thinly sliced
1 to 2 teaspoons curry powder
½ teaspoon ground cumin
¼ teaspoon ground cinnamon
Salt

In large saucepan fitted with steam basket, bring 2 inches water to a boil over high heat. Add sweet potatoes. Cover and cook until just tender, about 15 minutes (I just boil them, as I don't have a steamer).

Meanwhile, in another large saucepan, combine chickpeas, tomatoes, and ½ cup water. Bring to a simmer over medium heat. Add spinach, cover, and cook just until wilted, about 3 minutes.

Stir in sweet potatoes, cilantro, scallions, curry powder, cumin, cinnamon, and salt to taste until well combined. Reduce heat to low and simmer, uncovered, until flavors have blended, about 5 minutes. Serve hot.

Spicy Cold Soba Noodles
Susan Feniger and Mary Sue Milliken, a.k.a. "Two Hot Tamales"

SERVES 6

Marilu: *This is my favorite dish from the late, great City restaurant, whose cookbook (thank goodness) can still be found.*

I love this dish so much, I wanted to photograph it. There is a Zen quality that just makes me feel like I'm doing something great for my body.

Tasters' comments: *"Fantastic." "A+." "This is one of my three desert island choices."*

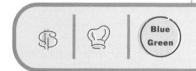

⅓ cup soy sauce

1 tablespoon molasses

¼ cup sesame oil

¼ cup tahini

1 tablespoon barley malt

¼ cup chili oil

3 tablespoons balsamic or red wine
   vinegar

½ bunch scallions, white and green
   parts, thinly sliced

Salt to taste

½ pound soba noodles (Japanese
   buckwheat noodles)

Place soy sauce in a pan over high heat and reduce by half. Turn heat to low, stir in molasses, and warm briefly. Transfer to a mixing bowl. Add sesame oil, tahini, barley malt, chili oil, vinegar, and scallions, and whisk to combine. Season to taste with salt, if desired.

Bring a large pot of salted water to a rapid boil. Add noodles, bring back to a boil, and cook, stirring occasionally, until they just begin to soften, about 3 minutes. (Soba noodles can overcook very quickly, so stay nearby.)

Have ready a large bowl of ice water. Drain noodles, plunge in ice water, and drain again. Place in a colander and rinse well under cold running water. Combine noodles and sauce, toss well, and chill.

Checca Pasta

Marilu: It's so easy to make and keeps well. Kids will love it.

Tasters' comments: "Oh my gosh, this is so fresh." "This would make a really nice summer pasta."

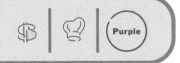

**10 to 12 plum tomatoes, peeled,
  seeded, and chopped**
10 to 12 basil leaves, chopped
3 cloves garlic, peeled and sliced thin

2 teaspoons olive oil
Salt and pepper
1 box pasta

No cooking time. Combine all the ingredients except the pasta 1 hour ahead to let the flavors combine. Cook any shape pasta until al dente. Toss with the sauce.

Pesto Primavera

SERVES 6

Tasters' comments: "So tasty and easy to make." "Very flavorful." "Great for kids because it has carbs and lots of veggies."

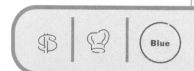

Pesto Sauce

2 cups fresh basil

¼ cup olive oil

2 tablespoons toasted pine nuts

1 clove garlic

Salt and pepper to taste

Sautéed Vegetables

2 cups broccoli florets

1 cup carrots, sliced

1 bunch asparagus tips

½ cup peas

¼ cup water

1 teaspoon soy margarine

Salt and pepper

1 box pasta

Blend pesto ingredients in food processor until well blended.

Sauté all vegetables in ¼ cup water with margarine for about 10 to 15 minutes. Season with salt and pepper.

Cook any shape pasta until al dente. Drain. Toss with pesto sauce and sautéed vegetables. Serve immediately.

Farfalle Funghi

Tasters' comments: *"The white beans make this so hearty." "This is a great cold-weather dish." "It would taste great with the mushrooms cut into chunks so they taste meaty."*

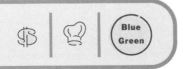

½ cup olive oil

2 large or 3 small cloves garlic

5 cups assorted mushrooms (porto-bello, chanterelle, oyster, shiitake, cremini)

8 fresh sage leaves, minced

1 can small white (navy) beans, drained

Salt and pepper to taste

1 box farfalle (bow-tie pasta)

Heat sauté pan. Add olive oil and garlic when it starts to sizzle. Add mushrooms and sage. Cook for 2 minutes. Add beans and cook on low heat for another 2 to 3 minutes. Season with salt and pepper.

Cook pasta according to box. Do not rinse. Drain and add to mushrooms and beans. Toss over very low heat.

Maria's Porcini Pasta with Pine Nuts

SERVES 4 TO 6

Marilu: We learned this dish from Maria, my friend from Italy, who could always whip up something incredible with what seemed like nothing from the cupboard.

Tasters' comments: "This has a creamy, woody Tuscan flavor."

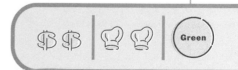

3 tablespoons olive oil

1 shallot

1 large or 2 small cloves garlic, minced

2 cups porcini mushrooms (you can buy dried porcinis and soak them to rehydrate)

Salt and pepper to taste

¼ cup pine nuts

1 box fusilli

¼ cup soy cream

Soy Parmesan

In a skillet over medium heat, warm olive oil. Add shallot, garlic, and mushrooms and cook for 3 minutes so flavors come together. Season with salt and pepper. Set aside.

In a toaster oven, toast half the pine nuts. Add both raw and toasted pine nuts to mushroom sauce.

Cook fusilli according to package instructions. Drain but do not rinse, so that sauce will stick. Toss with mushroom sauce. While tossing, add soy cream and soy Parmesan.

Butternut Squash Pasta

SERVES 4

Tasters' comments: *"What a great balance of sweet and hearty." "This is a perfect dish for any time of the year."*

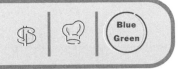

1 medium white onion, chopped

2 tablespoons soy margarine

1 pound butternut squash, peeled and
   cut into 2-inch pieces

¾ cup vegetable broth

1 teaspoon chopped sage

1 pound penne

2 tablespoons chopped Italian parsley

1 cup soy Parmesan

2 tablespoons soy margarine

Salt and freshly ground pepper

In a large skillet, cook onion with margarine over medium to high heat, stirring occasionally, until it's golden. Finely chop squash pieces in a blender or food processor and add to onion with vegetable broth. Simmer, covered, stirring occasionally, about 15 minutes, or until the squash is tender. Add the sage and simmer 1 more minute.

Cook the penne in a 6-quart pot of salted boiling water. Reserve 1 cup of the water and drain the pasta. Return pasta to a pot and add the squash mixture, parsley, soy Parmesan, soy margarine, and plenty of fresh ground pepper. Stir until the soy margarine is melted. Season with salt if necessary and add some of the reserved pasta-cooking water to moisten it if necessary.

White Bean Pasta

SERVES 4

Marilu: This delicious dish does something extraordinary: the white beans actually absorb the flavors of the sauce. It's a great combination with pasta.

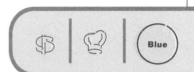

5 quarts water
½ pound ditalini pasta ("little thimbles")
2 tablespoons salt
Two 16-ounce cans white beans, drained

2 tablespoons olive oil
2 tablespoons soy margarine
2 teaspoons chopped fresh rosemary
1 very large or 2 medium-size onions, sliced paper thin
Freshly ground black pepper

In a soup kettle, bring the water to a boil. Add the pasta and the salt. Stir and continue to cook over high heat until the water returns to a boil. When the pasta is half cooked, about 6 minutes, add the beans to the pasta. While the pasta and the beans are cooking together, warm the oil and margarine in a skillet over medium heat. Add the rosemary and onion and sauté until lightly browned, about 10 minutes. When the pasta is al dente, drain it, and while it is still dripping, transfer it to a warm serving bowl. Add the browned onions and toss well. Sprinkle liberally with pepper to taste and more salt if desired. Serve at once.

Pine Nut and Marjoram Pasta

SERVES 4

Marilu: *When you're in the mood for that extra-creamy pasta, this is your flavor. Adult comfort food.*

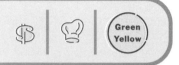

1 pound farfalle (bow-tie pasta)

10 tablespoons soy margarine

½ cup pine nuts, lightly toasted and roughly chopped

½ cup soy Parmesan

2 tablespoons chopped fresh marjoram

Freshly ground white pepper

Cook farfalle according to package directions.

Melt the soy margarine in a skillet large enough to accommodate the pasta. Drain the pasta, transfer to the skillet, and toss with margarine using two large forks, keeping the gentlest possible flame under the skillet. Distribute the margarine well through the pasta.

Add the pine nuts, soy Parmesan, marjoram, and pepper to taste and serve immediately.

Linguine with Pesto and Green Beans

SERVES 4

Marilu: This is a very hearty meal. It's an interesting flavor to have linguine with pesto contrasting with green beans.

Tasters' comments: "I recommend it."

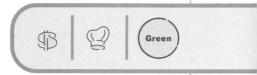

2 cups basil leaves

2 garlic cloves, peeled

2 teaspoons Bragg Liquid Aminos

¼ cup soy Parmesan

2 tablespoons olive oil

2 tablespoons soy margarine

2 tablespoons pine nuts

2 medium potatoes (about ½ pound), peeled and diced

1 pound linguine

½ pound string beans, trimmed and cut into 1-inch pieces

Salt

Bring a large pot of salted water to boil.

Combine the basil, garlic, Bragg's, and Parmesan in a blender or food processor. Pulse until roughly chopped. Add the olive oil and margarine and continue to blend until the mixture is fairly creamy, adding a little more olive oil if necessary. Add the pine nuts and pulse a few times to chop them in the sauce.

Add the potatoes to the boiling water and stir. Then add pasta and cook, stirring frequently, about 5 minutes. Add the string beans and cook about 5 minutes more, until pasta is done. When the pasta is done, the potatoes and beans should be tender. Drain the pasta and vegetables. Toss with pesto, adding more salt, Bragg's, and olive oil, if you like, and serve.

Pasta with White Beans and Rosemary

Elizabeth Carney

SERVES 4

Marilu: This pasta was a winner with the team. Lorin wanted to take the rest home. This is a nice combination of pasta and soup.

1⅓ cups (½ pound) dried cannellini or great Northern beans, or two 16-ounce cans white beans

½ pound shell pasta

1½ tablespoons salt

¼ cup extra-virgin olive oil

2 teaspoons chopped fresh rosemary, or 1 teaspoon dried rosemary

1 very large or 2 medium-size onions, sliced paper thin

4 cups vegetable stock

Freshly ground black pepper

If using dried beans, rinse and soak them overnight in 3 quarts of water. Cook for 1½ hours. Drain and set aside. If using canned beans, drain them, then rinse and drain well again; set aside.

In a soup kettle, bring 3 quarts water to a boil. Add the pasta and the salt. Continue to cook over high heat until the water returns to a boil, stirring frequently. When the pasta is half cooked (about 6 minutes), add the cooked beans to the pasta pot.

While the pasta and beans are cooking together, warm the oil in a skillet over medium heat. Add the rosemary and onion and sauté until lightly browned, about 10 minutes. When the pasta is al dente, drain it, and, while it is still dripping, transfer to a warmed serving bowl. Add the browned onion and toss well. Add warm vegetable stock until you reach a thick soup consistency.

Sprinkle liberally with pepper to taste and add more salt if desired. Then garnish with more chopped fresh rosemary and serve at once.

Caviar Pasta

Elizabeth Carney

SERVES 4

Elizabeth: When this pasta and caviar come together, it tastes like an entire plate of caviar.

Marilu: I wanted to lick the spoon.

Tasters' comments: "The two main ingredients combine to make a perfect texture." "It's a comfort food when you're feeling rich." "You'll want seconds."

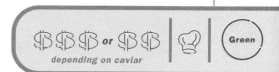

3 tablespoons olive oil
1 large shallot
1 clove garlic
½ cup vermouth
1 box pearl pasta (almost the shape of caviar, only larger)

2 tablespoons finely chopped fresh basil
1 tablespoon finely chopped fresh Italian parsley
2 ounces sevruga or osetra caviar

In a sauté pan, combine olive oil, shallot, garlic, and vermouth. Sauté at low heat until alcohol burns off. (Cooking at high temperature will cause the alcohol to flame.) Put sauce through fine strainer, and mush so that all juice comes out of shallots.

Cook pasta and drain. Toss with sauce. Add basil and parsley. Set on plates and top with dollop of caviar.

Note: Soy caviar is now available. If you use it, it will not only make the dish less expensive, but it will change it to a blue week recipe.

Side Dishes

Oven-Roasted Asparagus with Hazelnut Vinaigrette

Denise Barker

SERVES 2 TO 4

Denise: Fatter spears work well for this easy side dish. It's so delicious two people could happily share a portion this size.

Marilu: This totally yummy dish has a great combination of flavors. One of my boys actually said, "Please, sir, could I have some more?" This became a staff favorite.

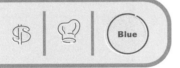

1 pound asparagus, trimmed

1 tablespoon olive oil

¼ teaspoon each salt and pepper

2 tablespoons minced shallots

2 tablespoons finely chopped toasted
   hazelnuts

1 tablespoon hazelnut or olive oil

1 tablespoon red wine vinegar

½ teaspoon Dijon mustard

Preheat oven to 500 degrees. Spread asparagus in a single layer on a large baking sheet. Drizzle with 1 tablespoon olive oil, then sprinkle with salt and pepper. Roast uncovered for about 8 minutes, turning once, or until asparagus is tender but still slightly firm.

Meanwhile, whisk together shallots, hazelnuts, hazelnut oil, vinegar, and mustard. Transfer hot asparagus to a warm platter and spoon dressing over the top. Toss gently to coat asparagus with dressing, then serve at once.

Green Beans with Pine Nuts

SERVES 6

Marilu: It has such a great flavor for such simple preparation.

Tasters' comments: "What a fabulous side dish." "The pine nuts really bring out the flavor of the beans."

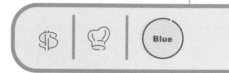

2 pounds young green beans, ends trimmed

1 tablespoon salt

2 tablespoons soy margarine

1 tablespoon extra-virgin olive oil

⅓ cup pine nuts, lightly toasted

In a saucepan, bring enough water to cover the beans to a rolling boil. Add the beans and salt. Cook until tender, about 6 to 7 minutes, then drain well. In a skillet over medium heat, melt the margarine with the oil. Add the beans and nuts to the pan, toss together, and serve at once.

Sautéed Broccoli Rabe

Marilu: *This succulent side dish really brings out the flavors in your meal. It's a great accent to fish and chicken.*

Tasters' comments: *"My favorite vegetable."*

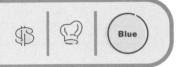

2 pounds broccoli rabe
1 tablespoon salt
1 tablespoon soy margarine
2 tablespoons extra-virgin olive oil

1 large garlic clove, cut in small
  pieces
Pinch of red pepper flakes

Using a small sharp paring knife, peel off the skin from the tough lower stalks of the rabe (most of the bottom portion of the stalk). Cut the rabe into approximately 3-inch lengths and wash it well. Fill a saucepan ¾ full of water and bring to a rolling boil. Drain the rabe and add the rabe and the salt to the pan. Cover partially and cook for 5 minutes after the water returns to a boil. Meanwhile, place the margarine, olive oil, garlic, and pepper flakes together in a cold skillet. Turn on the heat to low and sauté until the garlic starts to color, about 5 minutes. Do not let it brown.

Drain the rabe and transfer it to the skillet. Do not drain it so thoroughly that it is dry. It should be dripping somewhat from the transfer to the skillet. Stir covered and cook gently, stirring occasionally, until tender, about 5 minutes.

Green Beans with Roasted Onion

Beth Heffner

SERVES 12

Marilu: The roasted onion has a great texture with the crunchy green beans.

Tasters' comments: "The vinegar and Sucanat pull out so much sweetness." "Fabulous flavor."

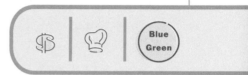

Vegetable oil spray
6 onions, peeled, each cut vertically
    into 12 to 14 wedges
6 tablespoons soy margarine
Salt and pepper to taste

2 cups vegetable broth
3 tablespoons Sucanat
2 tablespoons red wine vinegar
3 pounds French-style green beans,
    ends trimmed

Preheat oven to 450 degrees. Spray 2 large, heavy baking sheets with vegetable oil spray. Arrange onions in single layer on prepared sheets. Dot onions with 4 tablespoons soy margarine, dividing equally. Season with salt and pepper. Bake until onions are dark brown on bottom, about 35 minutes.

Boil broth in heavy large skillet over high heat until reduced to ½ cup, about 6 minutes. Add Sucanat and vinegar and whisk until Sucanat dissolves and mixture comes to a boil.

Add onions to sauce; reduce heat to medium-low. Simmer until liquid is slightly reduced, about 5 minutes. Season with salt and pepper. (Can be prepared 1 day ahead. Cover and refrigerate. Rewarm over low heat before continuing.)

Cook green beans in large pot of boiling salted water until crisp-tender, about 5 minutes. Drain well. Return beans to same pot. Add remaining 2 tablespoons soy margarine and toss to coat. Mound beans in large shallow bowl. Top with onion mixture and serve.

Steamed Spinach with Tarragon and Sesame Seeds

SERVES 4

Tasters' comments: *"Three of my favorite flavors together. Lots of iron and calcium. Healthy and tasty. You'll want to smile after you eat this, but check your teeth."*

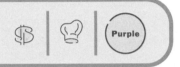

1 tablespoon salt

¼ bunch fresh tarragon

1 pound fresh spinach, cleaned, stems removed

Sesame seeds to sprinkle on top

Fill saucepan with water only up to steamer basket bottom. Add salt and tarragon to water. Add steamer basket with spinach. Cover and bring water to a boil for about 2 to 3 minutes. Turn off heat. Keep covered for an additional 1 to 2 minutes. Serve with sesame seeds sprinkled on top.

Brussels Sprouts with Vinegar-Glazed Onions

Beth Heffner

SERVES 4

Marilu: Don't just save it for a Christmas treat, it's too good.

Tasters' comments: "These were a big hit." "The perfect marriage of my two favorite vegetables." "A real holiday flavor."

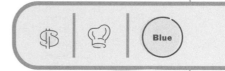

1 basket brussels sprouts
   (about 10 ounces)
Salt
1 tablespoon soy margarine
1 tablespoon olive oil

Freshly ground pepper
1 small red onion, thinly sliced
   lengthwise
2 tablespoons balsamic vinegar

Trim the outer leaves and stems from the brussels sprouts and discard. Bring a medium pot of water to a boil and add salt. Add brussels sprouts and cook until tender but still bright green, about 4 minutes. Remove from heat, drain, and plunge into a bowl of ice water to cool. Drain well and cut in half.

Heat ½ tablespoon soy margarine and ½ tablespoon olive oil in a large heavy skillet over medium-high heat. Add brussels sprouts and cook, tossing occasionally, until they are brown and crisp on the edges, about 3 minutes. Season to taste with salt and pepper and transfer to a large bowl. Cover with foil to keep warm.

Add remaining soy margarine and oil to the same pan over medium-low heat. Add the onions and cook, tossing occasionally, until wilted and transparent, about 3 to 4 minutes. Add the vinegar (stand back to avoid the fumes), and stir to loosen any brown bits on bottom of pan. Cook until vinegar is reduced and onions are glazed, about 30 seconds.

Add the onions to the brussels sprouts and toss well. Serve immediately.

Crunchy Coleslaw

Denise Barker

Marilu: *If you want to be a food-combining purist, leave out the raisins.*

Tasters' comments: *"This is one of my favorite flavors." "I'd like to try it without the raisins."*

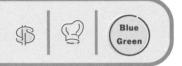

1 pound cabbage

¼ pound carrots

4 ounces raisins, washed and dried
   (optional if food combining)

4 ounces nuts of choice

Nayonaise

Shred or finely chop cabbage. Coarsely grate the carrots. Mix the cabbage, carrots, raisins, and nuts together in a large mixing bowl. Stir in enough Nayonaise to moisten the mixture. Chill. This looks nice served on a bed of lettuce.

Thai Coleslaw

Stephanie O'Driscoll

SERVES 4 TO 6

Stephanie: *This is very good and I adjust the ingredients every time. If you let it sit, it will release a lot of juice, so you only need a little dressing! It is also good for a late-night snack!*

Marilu: *It's coleslaw with a real kick!*

Tasters' comments: *"Wow, what great flavors." "This reminds me of a dish from a restaurant." "It's almost like a cucumber dish served with satay."*

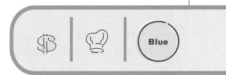

½ head green cabbage, shredded
½ head red cabbage, shredded
3 carrots, shredded
2 cups rice wine vinegar

⅛ teaspoon sesame oil
1½ teaspoons honey
1 teaspoon Thai hot sauce
2 teaspoons sesame seeds

Combine cabbage and carrots. In a separate bowl, combine vinegar, oil, honey, hot sauce, and sesame seeds. Toss and mix well with cabbage and carrots.

Mashed Potatoes

Marilu: Very flavorful side dish. Nice change from the traditional.

Tasters' comments: "These are creamy and oh, so good."

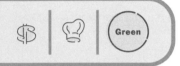

4 russet potatoes, peeled and cubed   **1 clove garlic, crushed**
½ cup soy cream cheese   **Salt and pepper**
2 tablespoons soy margarine

Cook potatoes in medium pot covered with water about 30 minutes. Drain. Mix with electric hand mixer. Add cream cheese, margarine, garlic, salt, and pepper. Keep warm.

Note: Reserve ¼ cup potato water to use if mixture is a little stiff. Add 1 tablespoon at a time.

Golden Mashed Potatoes and Arugula

SERVES 6

Marilu: I love the combination of arugula and chives.

Tasters' comments: "These are so good." "The added arugula gives it some extra bite."

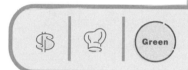

2½ pounds potatoes, well scrubbed, quartered, and skinned

1 bunch arugula, stems removed

1 cup Silk brand soy cream

1 tablespoon soy margarine

¼ teaspoon ground pepper

2 tablespoons minced chives

Salt to taste

In a large pot fitted with a steamer basket, bring 2 inches water to a boil. Put the potatoes in the basket. Reduce heat to medium, cover, and steam until the potatoes are very tender, 25 to 30 minutes.

Cut the arugula leaves crosswise into ¼ inch-thick strips. In a large bowl, combine the potatoes, Silk soy cream, soy margarine, and pepper. Using a potato masher, mash to a coarse puree. Stir in the arugula, chives, and salt to taste.

To serve, divide among individual plates.

Truffled Mashed Potatoes

SERVES 6 TO 8

Tasters' comments: *"This takes plain mashed potatoes and makes them gourmet."*
"These are so creamy and tasty."

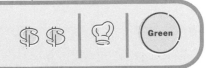

4 pounds white potatoes, peeled, cut
    into 1-inch pieces
1 cup soy creamer
¼ cup soy margarine
¼ cup olive oil

1 tablespoon white truffle oil
Salt and pepper
1 teaspoon shaved black truffles
    (optional)

Cook potatoes in large pot of boiling salted water until they are tender, about 20 minutes. Drain, return potatoes to pot. Stir over medium heat until moisture evaporates, about 1 minute. Remove from heat and add soy creamer, margarine, olive oil, and truffle oil. Mash until smooth. Season to taste with salt and pepper. Stir in truffles if desired.

Three-Grain Pilaf

Denise Barker

SERVES 4

Marilu: The wheat berries are so good for you. You'll probably burn as many calories chewing as you take in consuming.

Tasters' comments: "What a great texture."

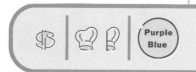

¼ cup hulled wheat berries
1 tablespoon olive oil
¼ cup wild rice
1½ cups water
¼ cup white wine
1 bay leaf
Salt and pepper to taste

¼ cup uncooked basmati rice
2 shallots, minced
1 cup (4 ounces) quartered shiitake
    mushrooms, stems removed
⅓ cup (2 ounces) chopped almonds
    with skins
4 green onions, thinly sliced

Soak wheat berries in enough water to cover for 2 hours, then drain. Put half the oil, the wheat berries, and the wild rice in a medium saucepan over medium heat and stir well. Add water, wine, bay leaf, and salt and pepper to taste. Bring to a boil. Cover, lower heat, and simmer 30 minutes. Stir in basmati rice.

Simmer, covered, 20 minutes longer. Remove from heat and allow to stand, covered. Heat remaining oil in large skillet and sauté shallots and shiitake mushrooms until softened, 3 to 4 minutes. Add almonds and cook, stirring, 3 to 4 minutes. Stir in green onions and cooked grains.

Pretty Herby Rice

Ruth A. Johnson

SERVES 4

Tasters' comments: *"This is a hearty fall or winter dish." "These flavors are great to-gether." "Might stick to your ribs, but cleans out your colon."*

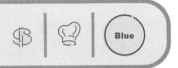

1 cup uncooked long-grain brown rice
14½ ounces vegetable broth
1 cup sliced zucchini
1 cup corn kernels
½ teaspoon pepper

1 teaspoon onion powder
1 clove garlic, minced
1 cup diced tomatoes
1 teaspoon dried basil

In medium saucepan, combine everything except tomatoes and basil. Cook over high heat until boiling. Reduce to low, cover, and simmer 15 to 20 minutes. Stir in tomatoes and basil; cook 10 to 15 minutes until heated through.

Leftover Mexican Rice and Rye

Donna Viola

SERVES 4

Donna: *Here is a recipe I use when I have made too much rice and rye.*

Marilu: *Great for those nights when you just want to toss something together.*

Tasters' comments: *"A healthy dish that is so satisfying."*

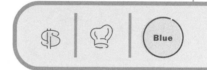

1 cup cooked rice and rye

1 cup cooked black beans

1 cup corn

1 cup salsa (mild or hot, for whatever mood you're in)

2 to 4 cups vegetable broth, depending on whether you want a soup or stew consistency

Mix all ingredients together in a saucepan and simmer 30 to 45 minutes, stirring occasionally.

Danielle's Spicy Rice and Rye with Veggies

Danielle Helmer

SERVES 2

Danielle: I came up with this using leftover rice and rye.

Marilu: You could make this as a main course meal and serve it with a salad.

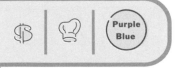

2 tablespoons light soy sauce

4 to 5 drops chili oil (Mongolian Fire Oil is really good)

½ tablespoon Dijon mustard

1 tablespoon Annie's Low-Fat Gingerly Dressing (or any healthy, low-fat salad dressing)

2 tablespoons chopped onion

2 tablespoons chopped white button mushroom caps

½ cup chopped zucchini

1 cup chopped broccoli

1½ cups prepared rice and rye

1 tablespoon chopped green onions

Cayenne pepper to taste

Wisk soy sauce, chili oil, Dijon mustard, and dressing together and add to medium saucepan over medium heat. Add onion and mushrooms and sauté for a few minutes. Add zucchini and broccoli and sauté for another 3 minutes. Add cooked rice and rye to vegetable mixture. Lastly, add chopped green onions and sprinkle with cayenne pepper.

Sauces

Tomato Basil Sauce

Tasters' comments: *"This is an extremely simple pasta sauce recipe that will impress even your Italian friends."*

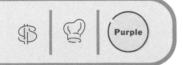

One 28-ounce can whole tomatoes, pureed

4 cloves garlic, crushed and chopped

4 teaspoons olive oil

10 to 12 basil leaves, chopped

Salt and pepper to taste

In a medium saucepan, combine all ingredients together. No sautéing needed. Cook 25 minutes. Toss with any cooked pasta.

Pomodoro Sauce

SERVES 4

Marilu: This simple sauce can be made and then stored for future use. Great on pasta for a last-minute meal.

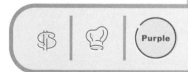

1 tablespoon olive oil

1 onion, chopped

2 cloves garlic, minced

1 can chopped or diced tomatoes

One 14-ounce can tomato sauce

1 cup sliced mushrooms (optional)

1 tablespoon basil (fresh preferred, but can use ½ tablespoon dried)

1 tablespoon oregano (fresh preferred, but can use ½ tablespoon dried)

In a saucepan, combine olive oil, onion, and garlic. Sauté until onions are translucent. Add chopped tomatoes, sauce, and mushrooms, if desired. Simmer on low 20 to 30 minutes, covered. Add basil and oregano. Serve over pasta.

My Not-So-Secret-Anymore Tomato Sauce

Ruth A. Johnson

MAKES ABOUT 3 CUPS

Ruth: I love this over whole wheat spaghetti. It also makes a great pizza sauce!

Marilu: A great all-purpose sauce.

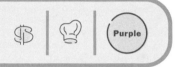

1 teaspoon olive oil

1 cup chopped onion

4 minced cloves garlic

2 tablespoons balsamic vinegar

1 tablespoon sweetener of choice (optional)

1 teaspoon dried basil

2 tablespoons tomato paste

½ teaspoon dried Italian seasoning

¼ teaspoon black pepper

Two 14.5-ounce cans diced tomatoes, with juices

2 tablespoons chopped fresh parsley

Heat oil in a saucepan over medium-high heat. Add onion and garlic; sauté 5 minutes. Stir in vinegar, sweetener, basil, tomato paste, Italian seasoning, pepper, and tomatoes and bring to a boil. Reduce to medium heat and cook, uncovered, about 15 minutes. Stir in parsley.

Lime Coconut Dressing

Denise Barker

Marilu: *A good combination for a mixed green salad. Serve with fish as a second course if you're not food combining.*

Tasters' comments: *"Tart and sweet."*

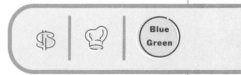

Juice of 3 to 4 limes

2 tablespoons olive oil

1 teaspoon chopped fresh basil

1 clove garlic, minced

1 teaspoon Sucanat

½ cup coconut milk

1 teaspoon dried chili flakes

Mix all dressing ingredients together. Can be stored up to one week in the fridge. Also, it can be used as a dressing for any salad.

Sweet and Sour Fruit Salad Dressing

Denise Barker

MAKES 1¾ CUPS DRESSING

Tasters' comments: "This is really versatile. It goes great with coleslaw, fresh fruit, Waldorf salad, or apple crumble pie."

½ pound firm tofu, mashed
¼ cup canola oil
¼ cup lemon juice
¼ cup honey

¼ teaspoon cinnamon
¼ teaspoon vanilla
⅛ teaspoon salt

Place all ingredients in a blender or food processor. Blend until smooth and creamy.

I have served this over fruit salad to company and received rave reviews.

Fresh Coriander Chutney

Denise Barker

MAKES APPROXIMATELY 1½ CUPS

Marilu: This is a tangy and delightful addition to fish or chicken. Also good on a salad.

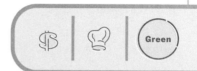

1 bunch (¼ pound) coriander (also known as cilantro), leaves and stems

¼ cup lemon juice

2 tablespoons water

¼ cup grated coconut

2 tablespoons chopped fresh ginger

1 teaspoon honey

1 teaspoon sea salt

¼ teaspoon freshly ground black pepper

Blend coriander, lemon juice, and water in a food processor or blender until chopped. Add the remaining ingredients and process until a paste forms. This can be stored in the fridge for up to 1 week. This is a fast chutney that tastes great on East Indian dishes.

Olive's Citrus Aioli

Todd English

MAKES ABOUT 1½ TO 2 CUPS

Todd: Citrus aioli is good on grilled fish, chicken, oysters, or shrimp. I like it in tuna salad instead of regular mayonnaise.

Marilu: Another great flavor from Olive's.

Tasters' comments: "Complicated flavors that go so well with fish."

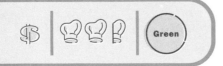

2 garlic cloves
Grated zest and juice of ½ lime
Grated zest and juice of ½ orange
Grated zest and juice of ½ lemon
½ cup fresh bread crumbs
2 large egg yolks
½ teaspoon Hungarian paprika

½ teaspoon kosher salt
½ teaspoon black pepper
1 tablespoon water
1¼ cups olive oil
¼ cup finely chopped fresh cilantro
   leaves
¼ cup finely chopped scallions

Place the garlic, citrus zest and juices, bread crumbs, egg yolks, paprika, salt, and pepper in a blender and process for 1 minute. Add the water and process to blend. While the machine is running, gradually add the oil in a thin, steady stream and process until smooth. Stir in the cilantro and scallions.

Soy Sour Cream or Cream Topping

Denise Barker

SERVES 4

Denise: This is great to put on top of crepes.

Marilu: Reminds me of crème fraîche.

Tasters' comments: "This is good on the palate." "Perfect when you need a sweet type of sour cream."

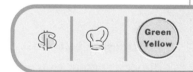

8 ounces firm tofu
¼ cup oil
1 tablespoon lemon juice

1½ teaspoons sugar or honey
½ teaspoon sea salt

Place all ingredients in blender and blend until mixed. To make cream topping, just add extra honey or sugar, whichever you prefer.

Mock Mayonnaise

Denise Barker

MAKES 1¼ CUPS

Marilu: This has a great consistency. It works well on veggie burgers or fish sandwiches. It adds a lot of flavor.

5 ounces firm tofu

3 ounces regular tofu or soft tofu

2 tablespoons lemon juice

1½ tablespoons Sucanat

1 clove garlic, minced

½ tablespoon almond butter

½ teaspoon salt

In a blender or food processor, blend all ingredients until smooth. Serve immediately or refrigerate and serve cold.

Homemade Garlic Mayonnaise

Ruth A. Johnson

MAKES JUST UNDER 1 CUP

Marilu: This sauce adds kick and zip to sandwiches and veggie burgers. Try it with Chicago Diner's Oatburgers (page 247).

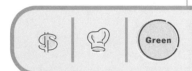

1 egg yolk

½ teaspoon Dijon mustard

Salt to taste

2 cloves garlic, minced

¾ cup olive oil

1 tablespoon lemon juice

Combine egg yolk, mustard, salt, and garlic. Whisk together. Gradually add oil. Once blended, add lemon juice. Keep refrigerated.

Champagne Vinaigrette

Tasters' comments: *"This decadent salad dressing is great on anything that needs a festive kick."*

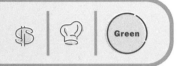

6 tablespoons champagne vinegar
½ cup almond oil

Whisk the vinegar into the oil.

Hazelnut Vinaigrette

Tasters' comments: *"This has a woodsy quality that is great to bring out the flavor of nuts in a salad."*

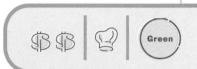

6 tablespoons white wine vinegar
½ cup hazelnut oil

Salt and freshly ground pepper to taste

Whisk the vinegar into the oil. Add salt and pepper according to personal taste.

Desserts

Coconut Sorbet

Denise Barker

MAKES 2 CUPS

Marilu: You won't miss ice cream with this dessert. It sure passes the kid test. Try it with almond extract as well.

Tasters' comments: "Yum, yum." "This is fantastic, it tastes like ice cream."

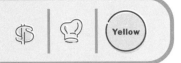

One 14-ounce can coconut milk
5 tablespoons fructose
Pinch sea salt

¼ teaspoon vanilla extract, or
¼ vanilla bean, scraped

In a bowl, combine all ingredients. Freeze in an ice cream maker according to manufacturer's instructions. If you do not have an ice cream maker, pour mixture into a shallow baking pan and place in a level area of your freezer. Freeze for 4 to 6 hours, stirring every hour, until mixture is frozen.

Note: Fructose is a natural by-product of fruit and honey, also called fruit sugar. You can purchase this in granulated or liquid form. This is easy to dissolve in liquids. You could also try substituting 6 tablespoons of honey, maple, or rice syrup.

Mexican-Style Rice Pudding

Heather Anderson

SERVES 4

Heather Anderson: *I've gone from a size 16 to an 8 since starting your program approximately 1 year ago. My life has totally turned around, because I also confronted the emotional issues that were largely responsible for the weight gain in the first place. I also recruited my best friend to dump dairy, sugar, and caffeine, and we are both running the L.A. marathon next month. Talk about a before-and-after photo op! Thanks.*

Tasters' comments: *"I love this." "Make it without the raisins to food-combine." "This is sweet, but not too sweet." "What a great texture, like a moist chewiness." "My kind of dessert."*

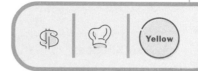

2½ cups vanilla-flavored rice milk
  (use soy milk for creamier texture)
2 cups cooked white or brown rice
  (add more milk for brown rice)
¼ cup Sucanat or other sugar substitute (amount varies according to sweetener used—recipe originally called for ½ cup of sugar, and Sucanat tastes pretty concentrated to me, so I reduced by half)

¼ cup raisins (bad combining, I know!)
¼ cup grated unsweetened coconut (I love coconut, so I add more, usually ½ cup)
1 teaspoon vanilla extract
1 whole cinnamon stick
One 4-inch strip of lime or orange peel

In a medium saucepan, combine all ingredients. Cook over medium-low heat, stirring frequently, until the rice is thick and the fruit is slightly tender, about 30 minutes. Remove from heat and let cool slightly. Transfer to a bowl and refrigerate at least 1 hour before serving.

When ready to serve, discard the cinnamon stick and citrus peel. Spoon into bowls and serve. If desired, garnish each bowl with a twist of lime or orange peel.

Carrot Spice Cookies

Deryn Collier

MAKES 18 TO 24 COOKIES

Deryn: My big pitfall is cookies and baked things, but with recipes like this, quitting sugar should be a piece of cake! (Sugar free, of course!!)

Tasters' comments: "What a perfect food combination with a lot of flavor." "This is perfect when you want something sweet and to stay within the rules."

½ cup Sucanat
½ cup maple syrup
½ cup soy milk
3 tablespoons sesame seeds
2 tablespoons oil
1 teaspoon vanilla
1 cup grated carrots (about 4 to 5 small)

1 teaspoon grated fresh ginger
1¼ cup whole wheat flour
½ cup soy, amaranth, or brown rice flour
1 teaspoon baking powder
¼ teaspoon salt
½ teaspoon cinnamon
¼ teaspoon nutmeg

Mix the first 8 ingredients (through the ginger) in a bowl. In a separate bowl, mix all the remaining ingredients. Preheat oven to 325 degrees. Gradually beat Sucanat mixture into flour mixture until well mixed. Dollop with teaspoon onto oiled baking sheets. Bake for 15 minutes or until golden brown.

Pumpkin Cookies

Denise Barker

Tasters' comments: *"Healthy-tasting and good-flavored cookie that doesn't weigh you down."*

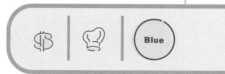

¾ cup honey

1 cup pumpkin puree

½ cup oil

1 teaspoon vanilla

2 cups flour of choice

¼ cup soya flour

2½ teaspoons baking powder

½ teaspoon salt

1 teaspoon cinnamon

½ teaspoon nutmeg

¼ teaspoon ginger

1 cup raisins (optional)

½ cup chopped nuts (optional)

Preheat oven to 350 degrees. Mix honey, pumpkin, oil, and vanilla in a bowl. In a separate bowl, combine dry ingredients; add to pumpkin mix. Stir in raisins and nuts, if desired. Drop by spoonfuls onto oiled cookie sheet. Bake for 12 to 15 minutes.

Our Favorite Chocolate Chip Cookies

Elizabeth Carney

MAKES 8 DOZEN 2-INCH COOKIES

Marilu: *Great for snack day at school. My niece brings them to parties and no one knows the difference between dairy and non-dairy.*

Tasters' comments: *"These are great even for non–chocolate lovers." "These are so so good, they taste like the real thing."*

   Green Yellow

2¼ cups unsifted all-purpose flour
1 level teaspoon baking soda
1 level teaspoon salt
1 cup soy margarine
1 cup Sucanat
½ cup date sugar
1 teaspoon vanilla extract

2 large eggs
One 12-ounce package semisweet non-dairy chocolate chips (such as Tropical Source)
½ cup chopped nuts (optional)
½ cup raisins (optional)

Preheat oven to 375 degrees. In a small bowl, combine flour, baking soda, and salt. Set aside. In larger bowl, combine soy margarine, Sucanat, date sugar, and vanilla extract; beat until creamy. Beat in eggs, one at a time. Gradually add flour mixture. Mix well before stirring in non-dairy chocolate chips. Add nuts and raisins at this time, if desired.

Drop rounded teaspoonfuls of dough onto ungreased cookie sheets. Bake for 8 to 10 minutes.

Nicky and Joey's Cookies

Donna Erickson

MAKES 18 TO 24 COOKIES

Donna: We made these cookies for the boys' school snack, and all of the kids loved them.

Marilu: Every time she made them, the whole team ate them before they cooled.

Tasters' comments: "The boys love them."

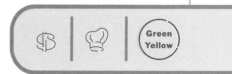

1½ cups maple sugar
½ cup soy margarine
3 ounces soft tofu
5 tablespoons unsweetened apple-
    sauce
2 tablespoons egg whites (from
    about 1 egg)
1 teaspoon vanilla extract

2 cups oat flour
½ teaspoon baking powder
½ teaspoon baking soda
½ teaspoon sea salt
2 cups quick-cooking rolled oats
¾ cup non-dairy peanut butter
    chocolate chips
Canola oil spray

Preheat the oven to 375 degrees. In a mixing bowl, mix together the maple sugar, soy margarine, tofu, and applesauce thoroughly. Add the egg whites and vanilla and mix.

In another mixing bowl, sift together the flour, baking powder, baking soda, and salt. Add the oats and mix thoroughly. Add the dry ingredients to the wet mixture, and lightly blend with a plastic spatula. Add the peanut butter chocolate chips and stir with the spatula to mix.

Spray a nonstick cookie sheet with canola oil spray. Put teaspoon-size dollops of the dough on the cookie sheet. Bake for 12 to 15 minutes, until golden brown. Store up to 10 days in an airtight container.

Sesame Sweeties

Denise Barker

MAKES 1 DOZEN

Marilu: "Mmmm, good."

Tasters' comments: "This not too sweet confection has a great flavor." "A sesame and coconut lover's dream."

½ cup sesame seeds

⅓ cup honey

2 tablespoons raw sunflower seeds

2 tablespoons tahini or sesame butter

½ cup sunflower seeds

⅛ teaspoon sea salt

1 teaspoon vanilla extract

½ cup unsweetened shredded coconut

Grind sesame seeds into powder in a food processor, grinder, or blender. In a mixing bowl, combine ground seeds with all other ingredients except coconut until they form a stiff and slightly crumbly dough. Press into 12 balls and roll in coconut. Chill for ½ hour.

Must-Have Macaroons

MaryAnn Hennings

MAKES 12

Marilu: Moist and delicious. Taste like the sinful kind.

Tasters' comments: "Phenomenal." "Amazing." "A++." "These have so much flavor."

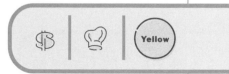

3 egg whites

Pinch of salt

¾ cup Sucanat

13 ounces coconut, grated

Preheat oven to 350 degrees. In a medium-size bowl, beat egg whites until stiff, gradually adding salt and Sucanat. By hand, blend in coconut.

Drop large tablespoons of dough onto an ungreased cookie sheet. Bake for 20 minutes.

Cool on waxed paper.

Killer Brownies

MaryAnn Hennings

Marilu: Great treat.

Tasters' comments: "These brownies are my favorite of all." "What a perfect dessert."
"This passes the kid test with flying colors." "All of the flavor of junk food and none of the junk."

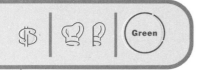

4 ounces unsweetened chocolate

1 cup soy margarine

1¾ cups Sucanat or maple sugar

4 large eggs

1 tablespoon vanilla extract

1 cup unbleached all-purpose flour

½ teaspoon salt

½ cup chopped walnuts (optional)

Preheat oven to 325 degrees. Lightly grease and flour a 9 x 9 or 8 x 8-inch baking pan.

Over the lowest possible heat, melt chocolate and soy margarine in a small saucepan, stirring occasionally. Set aside to cool to room temperature.

Combine the Sucanat, eggs, and vanilla in a medium-size mixing bowl. Whisk together until slightly frothy. Add cooled chocolate mixture and mix until just combined. Add flour and salt and mix until well combined. Add walnuts, if desired, and mix.

Place batter in pan and bake for about 25 to 30 minutes, or until a tester comes out clean.

Chocolate Mousse

Chicago Diner

Marilu: There is a chocolate god!!

Tasters' comments: "This is fantastic." "I'd love it on brownies." "It will have chocolate lovers screaming everywhere, 'Now I know I can do this program!'"

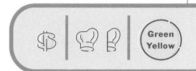

2 cups non-dairy chocolate chips, melted (We recommend naturally sweetened Sunspire chocolate chips)

1 box soft tofu, drained (approximately 12.5 ounces)
¾ cup soy milk
1 tablespoon maple syrup

Melt chocolate chips in a double boiler, or Pyrex dish over a pan of boiling water. Then place all ingredients in blender or food processor and process until smooth. Mixture will set in refrigerator after cooling 1 hour or more.

Serving Suggestions

1. Pour into parfait glasses or serving dishes for individual mousses and refrigerate.
2. Double the recipe, pour into prebaked pie shell, and refrigerate.
3. Refrigerate until firm and use in place of frosting for cakes.

Chocolate Graham Cracker Pudding Pie

Barb Conaway

Marilu: Joey had a friend (a sugar and dairy lover) over after we had tested this recipe and I gave it to them for a snack. He wanted seconds. This is so good, I can't believe it's on the program.

Crust

One 12-ounce box chocolate whole wheat graham crackers (such as New Morning brand)

¾ cup melted soy margarine or maple syrup

Filling

2 packages (4 ounces each) Mori Nu Mates chocolate pudding mix (or other non-dairy pudding mix)

2 packages firm low-fat silken tofu (to make pie filling as directed on Mori Nu package)

Break graham crackers into bite-size pieces and blend in a food processor until they are coarse crumbs. Transfer them to a mixing bowl. Slowly add the melted margarine or maple syrup and mix with hands until crumbs can be molded into a ball. Press about ¾ of the crumbs firmly into a lightly oil-sprayed 9-inch pie pan to form the bottom and sides. (Reserve remaining ¼ of the crumbs for the topping.)

Make the chocolate pudding according to the directions for a pie. Put it in the pie crust using a spatula and spread evenly to make it level.

Sprinkle the rest of the graham cracker crumbs on top and press gently to set. Refrigerate at least 4 hours or overnight.

Decadent Chocolate Cake

SERVES 6

Tasters' comments: *"This proves that chocolate lovers don't have to give up their chocolate."*

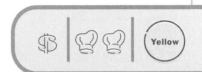

1 cup boiling water

3 ounces dairy-free chocolate (any Tropical Source kind is good)

8 tablespoons soy margarine

1 teaspoon vanilla extract

1 cup Sucanat

2 eggs, separated

1 teaspoon baking soda

1 cup soy sour cream

2 cups minus 2 tablespoons un-bleached all-purpose flour, sifted

1 teaspoon baking powder

Chocolate Frosting

5 tablespoons soy margarine

¾ cup non-dairy semisweet chocolate chips

6 tablespoons silk soy cream

1¼ cups fructose

1 teaspoon vanilla extract

Preheat oven to 350 degrees. Grease and flour a 10-inch tube pan.

Pour boiling water over chocolate and soy margarine; let stand until melted. Stir in vanilla and Sucanat, then whisk in egg yolks, one at a time.

Mix baking soda and sour cream and whisk into chocolate mixture. Sift flour and baking powder together and add to batter, mixing thoroughly. Beat egg whites until stiff but not dry. Stir a quarter of the egg whites thoroughly into the batter. Scoop remaining egg whites on top of the batter and gently fold together.

Pour batter into the prepared pan. Bake for 40 to 50 minutes, or until the edges have pulled away from the sides of the pan and a cake tester comes out clean. Cool in pan for 10 minutes; unmold and cool completely before frosting.

Place all frosting ingredients in a heavy saucepan over low heat and whisk until smooth. Cool slightly; add more fructose if necessary to achieve a spreading consistency. Spread on cake while frosting is still warm.

Orange Cake with Carob Glaze

Robin Papa

MAKES 1 CAKE

Robin: I converted this recipe to an acceptable THM one for my forty-sixth birthday. I was on day 10 of the Blue Book and didn't want to have to go back to boot camp! (Can anyone relate?)

I am certain that this will help me feel better, but even if it doesn't at least I'll know I'm my B.E.S.T. self!!!!! Be well and happy.

Marilu: We made this three times because we liked it so much.

Tasters' comments: "This reminds me of a rum cake." "What great, subtle flavor." "This could fool the nonbelievers." "All the testers ate it in one sitting." "Wow, so light and delicious." "Bring it to the table before cutting into it." "It's just like a sinful Bundt cake."

Green Yellow

Cake

3 eggs (or acceptable substitute)

2 cups vanilla-flavored soy yogurt

1½ teaspoons vanilla extract

2½ cups whole wheat flour, sifted to remove bran

⅔ cup unsweetened dried coconut (you can substitute ground almonds, I'm allergic to nuts)

1 cup Sucanat

1½ teaspoons baking powder

1 teaspoon baking soda

¾ teaspoon salt

2 tablespoons grated orange rind

1 cup soy margarine

Syrup

½ cup Sucanat

¼ cup fresh orange juice

Glaze

½ cup vanilla-flavored soy milk

⅔ cup carob chips (or dairy-free, grain-sweetened chocolate chips)

Preheat oven to 350 degrees. Spray a Bundt pan with cooking spray and dust with flour.

In a small bowl, lightly beat eggs, soy yogurt, and vanilla and set aside.

On low speed in the bowl of a mixer, stir sifted flour, coconut, Sucanat, baking powder, baking soda, salt, and orange rind for 30 seconds to blend. Add margarine and beat on low speed until dry ingredients are moistened, then beat at medium speed for 1½ minutes. Scrape bowl and add egg mixture. Beat for 1 more minute. Pour into pan and bake for 30 to 35 minutes or until cake tester comes out clean.

Meanwhile, make the syrup. Heat Sucanat and orange juice in saucepan until Sucanat is dissolved. Set aside to cool. To make the glaze, heat soy milk to very hot but not boiling and pour over carob chips. Stir until chips are melted and glaze is smooth.

When cake is done, place the pan on a cooling rack and brush the top with half of the orange syrup while the cake is hot. Wait 10 minutes and invert the cake on the rack to remove it from the pan. Spoon chocolate glaze over top of cake.

When cake is cool, place it on a serving plate and spoon the glaze over it so it drizzles down the sides.(If the glaze is too thick, you may have to warm it in the microwave slightly first.)

Maple Tofu Pie

Aaron Moskowitz

Aaron: Hello! My name is Aaron Moskowitz, and my aunt converted me into a healthy person by giving me your Total Health Makeover. I am 15 years old, and I was diagnosed with cancer over a year ago. I am now in remission and feel better than ever! I am so glad that I tried your program. Now I am healthier and happier than I have ever been, and I will follow your program forever! Here is a very good dessert recipe for maple tofu pie.

Marilu: I love the lightness of the flavor and the satisfaction of the sweetness.

Tasters' comments: "This is like a maple flan." "It looks so visually pleasing."

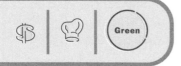

**1½ pounds firm or soft tofu, drained
   well**
¼ cup light canola oil
1⅓ cups real maple syrup

1 teaspoon vanilla
Pinch of salt
1 unbaked pie crust (see next recipe)

Preheat oven to 350 degrees. Break the tofu into pieces, then place in a blender or food processor with the rest of the pie ingredients and blend or process until smooth. Pour into the pie crust and bake for about 1 hour or until set. Chill and serve.

Whole Wheat Graham Cracker Crust

Ruth A. Johnson

Marilu: Try it with a fruit filling.

Tasters' comments: "This goes fabulously with the maple tofu pie." "A great base for any pie."

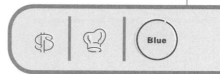

1½ cups whole wheat graham
   cracker crumbs

2 tablespoons soy margarine
2 tablespoons honey

Mix all ingredients and press into 9-inch pie pan. Bake at 350 degrees for about 8 minutes.

Tofu Cheesecake

Chicago Diner

Marilu: *A cheesecake lover's dream that even has a golden-brown topping.*

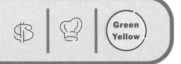

Crust

2 cups granola, graham cracker crumbs, or cookie crumbs

2 tablespoons soy margarine, melted

1 tablespoon water

Filling

1 tub soft silken tofu

1 tub firm silken tofu (12 to 14 ounces), drained

2 to 3 teaspoons lemon juice

1 cup maple syrup, honey, or Sucanat

⅓ cup canola oil or light vegetable oil

½ teaspoon salt

1 teaspoon vanilla extract

2 teaspoons lemon zest

1 cup non-dairy chocolate chips, chopped dried fruit, or coconut (optional)

Preheat oven to 350 degrees.

Crumble granola for crust with blender or food processor. Mix in melted margarine and water. If still very crumbly, add an additional tablespoon of water. Press mixture firmly into a 9-inch springform pan or pie pan. Bake for 10 to 15 minutes, checking periodically (ovens vary). Prepare filling as crust bakes.

Place all filling ingredients in a blender or food processor and process until smooth. If adding optional ingredients, fold into mixture now. Pour filling into crust and bake for 25 minutes. Check to see if top of cheesecake springs back at a light touch. If not, cook for an additional 5 to 10 minutes. Cool completely before slicing. Cheesecake will become firmer as it cools.

Note: For a larger cheesecake, double the recipe. For an even lower-cal recipe, use low- or no-fat granola and light tofu.

Silky Strawberry Pie

Elizabeth Carney

MAKES 1 PIE

Marilu: This has a great flavor and it's one of those desserts that looks too good to be true. If you are a fan of strawberries, you'll love it.

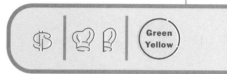

1 cup strawberries, cut in quarters, plus a few sliced thinly for garnish

2 tablespoons Sucanat

12 ounces extra-firm silken tofu

6 ounces firm silken tofu

2 tablespoons maple syrup

¼ teaspoon vanilla extract

1 baked graham cracker crust (see page 315)

Combine strawberries and Sucanat in a bowl and let sit for 5 minutes, or until a juice forms. In a food processor, blend the tofu, syrup, and vanilla until whipped. Add strawberry mixture and blend until smooth and a nice pink color. Fold into pie crust. Garnish with sliced strawberries. Refrigerate until set.

Chocolate Mousse Pie

Ruth A. Johnson

Marilu: This was a genuine hit. Love the bananas. Our New York friend compared it to a chocolate banana cream pie from a deli.

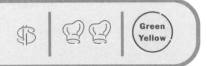

21 ounces firm silken tofu

1 cup non-dairy dark chocolate, melted

¾ cup unsweetened peanut butter (or other nut butter of choice)

2 tablespoons maple syrup (optional, for added richness)

1 baked graham cracker crust (see page 315)

1 or 2 ripe bananas

In a food processor or blender, blend the tofu, chocolate, and peanut butter. Add the maple syrup if desired. Line the piecrust with sliced banana. Pour the tofu mixture into the crust. Chill for at least 2 hours, or overnight.

appendix

HEALTHY LIFE SHOPPING LIST

Vegetables
Arugula
Avocados
Broccoli
Cabbage
Carrots
Celery
Cucumbers
Garlic, fresh
Ginger
Green beans, frozen
Mixed greens
Mushrooms, assorted
Onions (white, red, yellow)
Peas
Red cabbage
Scallions
Shallots
Spinach
Tomatoes (vine and plum)
Zucchini

Spices
Basil
Black pepper
Chervil
Cilantro
Cinnamon
Cumin
Crushed red pepper
Dill
Italian parsley
Oregano
Paprika
Parsley
Rosemary
Sea salt

Tarragon
Vanilla extract

Fruit and Juice
Apples
Grapes
Honeydews
Lemons
Limes
Seasonal fruit

Legumes
Black beans
Edamame (soy beans)
Great Northern beans (white)
Lentils
Pinto beans

Grains, Breads, Pasta
Brown Rice
Cereal (Puffins, Shredded
    Spoonfuls, Oatios, etc.)
Flourless whole-grain bread
    (Ezekiel 4:9ww)
Oatmeal
Pasta
Rye berries

Protein
Ahi tuna
Canned tuna
Eggs (cage-free)
Salmon
Swordfish steaks

Miscellaneous
Balsamic vinegar

Basmati rice
Bragg Liquid Aminos
Canola oil
Capers
Catsup (fruit juice–
    sweetened)
Dijon mustard
Extra-virgin olive oil
Herb teas
Honey
Light soy sauce
Maple sugar
Maple syrup
Miso
Miso soup
Mustard (fruit juice–
    sweetened)
Nayonaise
Olive oil spray
Red wine vinegar
Relish
Rice Dream
Salad dressing (Newman's
    Own Balsamic, Annie's
    Wild Herbal Organic)
Soy cheese
Soy margarine (Earth
    Balance)
Soy milk
Soy Parmesan (nonhydro-
    genated)
Sucanat
Sun-dried tomatoes
Tamari
Tofu (firm and extra-firm)
Vegetable stock or concen-
    trate

VEGETABLE SERVINGS

Vegetable	Serving for 2	Serving for 4
Artichoke	1 to 1½ pounds	2 to 2½ pounds
Asparagus	1 to 1½ pounds	2 to 2½ pounds
Beets	1 to 1½ pounds	2 to 2½ pounds
Bell peppers	1 pound	2 pounds
Broccoli	1 to 1½ pounds	2 to 2½ pounds
Brussels sprouts	¾ pound	1½ pounds
Cabbage	¾ pound	1½ pounds
Carrots	½ pound	1 pound
Cauliflower	1 ¼ pounds	2½ pounds
Corn on the cob	2 to 4 ears	8 ears
Eggplant	1 to 1½ pounds	2 to 2½ pounds
Green beans and string beans	1 to 1½ pounds	2 to 2½ pounds
Leeks	1 pound	2 pounds
Lima beans	1 to 1½ pounds	2 to 2½ pounds
Mushrooms	¾ pound	1½ pounds
Onions	1 pound	2 pounds
Peas	1 to 1½ pounds	2 to 2½ pounds
Potatoes	1 pound	2 pounds
Spinach	1 to 1½ pounds	2 to 2½ pounds
Squash	¾ pound	1½ pounds
Sweet potatoes	1 pound	2 pounds
Swiss chard	1 to 1½ pounds	2 to 2½ pounds
Zucchini	¾ pound	1½ pounds

GRAINS PRIMER

Grain	Description	Cooking Instructions
Amaranth	An Aztec grain with a sticky texture. Great in combination with other grains.	Cook 1 cup amaranth in 2½ cups water for 20 minutes. Yields 3 cups.
Barley	Beige kernels with extremely mild flavor and soft texture. Great as a side dish or added to soup.	Cook 1 cup barley in 2 cups water for 15 minutes. Yields 3 cups.
Buckwheat	Whole kernels with an earthy flavor. Roasted buckwheat is kasha and makes a great pilaf.	Cook 1 cup buckwheat in 2 cups water for 15 minutes. Yields 2½ cups.
Cornmeal	White or yellow corn kernels ground to a grainy powder. Sweet. Great in breads.	Cook 1 cup cornmeal in 4 cups water for 30 minutes. Yields 4 cups.
Millet	Small, light brown, whole kernels. Chewy and served like rice.	Cook 1 cup millet in 4 cups water for 30 minutes. Yields 4 cups.
Oats	Whole oat grain; nutty flavor and chewy texture. Wonderful breakfast food. Major claims of lowering cholesterol.	Cook 1 cup oats in 4 cups water for 60 minutes. Yields 4 cups.
Quinoa	Light yellow seed about the size of rice. Sweet flavor and soft texture. A whole protein in itself. Great as a salad base.	Cook 1 cup quinoa in 2 cups water for 15 minutes. Yields 3 cups.
Rice (brown)	Dark rice that is sweet and has hints of nut. Always a wonderful side dish.	Cook 1 cup brown rice in 2 cups water for 60 minutes. Yields 3 cups.
Rye berries	Small brown seedlike berries. A chewy grain that sucks the fat right out of your body (in my opinion). This is used in the rice and rye staple.	Cook 1 cup rye berries in 2½ cups water for 25 minutes. Yields 3 cups.
Wheat berries	Unprocessed whole-wheat kernels. Slightly chewy and great for baking.	Cook 1 cup wheat berries in 3 cups water for 2 hours. Yields 3 cups.
Wild rice	Long dark or light kernels with an earthy flavor.	Cook 1 cup wild rice in 2½ cups water for 50 minutes. Yields 3 cups.

BEANS AND LEGUMES PREPARATION TIPS

An important part of dried bean preparation is the preliminary soaking. Every bean with the exception of split peas and lentils should be soaked thoroughly before cooking. It is optimal to soak them overnight, but if it's not possible, try to soak larger, denser beans for 8 hours or more and smaller beans for at least 4 hours.

After picking through the dried beans and removing any withered ones, cover them with cold water and remove any beans that float to the top. Rinse as many times as needed to leave the water clear.

Note: Cooking times vary. The following are suggestions. You should really cook until beans are tender or to your liking. The water amounts are suggestions as well. The water will be discarded after the beans are cooked, so it's not essential to have measurements exact.

Bean	Description	Cooking Instructions
Adzuki	Small, oval, dark red beans. They have a nutlike flavor and light texture. Easily digestable.	Cook 1 cup dried beans in 4 quarts water for 1 hour and 15 minutes. Yields 2 cups.
Black	Medium-size oval beans. Soft texture. Great in soups.	Cook 1 cup dried beans in 3 quarts water for 1½ hours. Yields 2 cups.
Black-eyed peas	Small white bean with one black spot (the eye). A mealy texture. Great in stuffings and soups.	Cook 1 cup dried beans in 2¼ quarts water for 1 hour. Yields 2 cups.
Cannellini	Just like a white kidney bean. A nutty flavor. Prominently used in many Italian dishes.	Cook 1 cup dried beans in 1 quart water for 1½ to 2 hours. Yields 2 cups.
Fava (Broad)	Lightish brown in color, flat and kidney-shaped. Wonderful pureed. Remove the skins after cooking.	Cook 1 cup dried beans in 4 quarts water for 1½ hours. Yields 2 cups.
Garbanzo (Chickpeas)	Tan and round. They have a really hearty flavor. Used to make hummus and enhance the flavor of soups and salads.	Cook 1 cup dried beans in 4 quarts water for 2 to 3 hours. Yields 2 cups.
Kidney	Red bean with a kidney shape. Used in chili, salads, soups, and stews.	Cook 1 cup dried beans in 2 quarts water for 2 hours. Yields 2 cups.

Bean	Description	Cooking Instructions
Lentils	Many varieties. Shaped like tiny disks. The most common are red, brown, and green. Commonly used in Middle Eastern dishes.	Cook 1 cup dried beans in 4 cups water for 1 hour. Yields 2¾ cups.
Lima	Light green in color and flat. They come large and small and have a starchy texture.	Cook 1 cup dried beans in 2 quarts water for 1 ½ hours. Yields 2¾ cups.
Navy	Small and white. Very versatile. Slightly granular texture.	Cook 1 cup dried beans in 3½ quarts water for 1½ to 2 hours. Yields 2 cups.
Pinto	Large oval bean with a brown skin. Earthy flavor. Commonly in Spanish, Mexican, and southwestern dishes.	Cook 1 cup dried beans in 2 quarts water for 1½ to 2 hours. Yields 2 cups.
Red	Dark red and medium-size ovals. Similar to kidney beans. Used in many Mexican dishes.	Cook 1 cup dried beans in 2 quarts water for 1½ to 2 hours. Yields 2 cups.
Soybeans	Light green oval-like beans that come in a pea pod. One of the earth's most nutritious foods. Used to make tofu and miso.	Cook 1 cup dried beans in 3½ quarts water for 3 to 4 hours. Yields 2 cups.
Split peas	Small beans that come in yellow and green. Can be split or used whole. Great in soups.	Cook 1 cup dried beans in 4 cups water for 40 to 50 minutes. Yields 2 cups.
White (Great Northern)	Large and white with a grainy texture. Good in stews and hearty dishes.	Cook 1 cup beans in 3½ quarts water for 1 hour and 15 minutes. Yields 2 cups.

ADDING DRY HERBS AND SPICES

Just a touch of lemon juice brings out the flavors of the herbs in blending. Fresh herbs lose their flavor when cooked for a long time; add them later in the cooking process for optimal flavor.

Food	Herb/Spice Combination
Fish	Bay leaf and basil
	Rosemary and tarragon
	Mint, chervil, and fennel
Free-range chicken	Marjoram and Italian parsley
	Basil, bay, and thyme
	Rosemary and tarragon
Meat substitutes	Thyme, summer savory, sweet basil, and coriander (just a few seeds)
	Chervil, rosemary, sage, and savory
	Tarragon and basil
Pasta	Italian parsley, thyme, and garlic powder
	Basil, bay leaf, and oregano
Rice	Chervil and mint
	Marjoram, chervil, and savory
Salads	Basil and rosemary
	Mint and dill
Soup	Basil, rosemary, and savory
	Rosemary and marjoram

glossary

Ahi Tuna High-grade, meaty tuna, generally cut into steaks for broiling, grilling, or baking. Found in the fresh fish section or fish market.

Arborio Rice A hard-grain rice used in risotto and harvested in northern Italy. Found in the grain section.

Arugula Also known as rocket, roquette, rugula. A leafy lettuce with a distinct, peppery bite. Found in the produce section.

Balsamic Vinegar A vinegar aged from Trebbiano grapes. It is both sweet and sour, sometimes aged and sometimes quickly fermented, then aged. Wonderful with salad dressings. Prices range due to amount of aging. Found in the condiment section.

Bok Choy This popular vegetable in China is a small plant with dark green leaves on flat white stalks. It is sweet, crisp, and mild. Found in the produce section.

Bragg Liquid Aminos All-purpose liquid seasoning made from vegetable protein. Great for salads, salad dressings, stir-fries, soups, fish, and so on. Found in the health food section or health food stores.

Burdock Root Tea A caffeine-free tea from the burdock plant that aids in digestion and promotes weight loss. Found at health food stores.

Capers When pickled, these bulletlike buds of the caper bush taste like tiny sharp gherkins. Use them in tartar sauce, with fish, whenever you want a piquant note. They are both tart and salty. Found in the condiment section.

Cereal (Puffins, Shredded Spoonfuls, Oatios) Three great sugarless cereals made by Barbara's Bakery. They can generally be purchased at any health food store.

Chamomile An herb related to the daisy family. It is usually used as a tea to calm and relieve stress and anxiety. Found in the tea section.

Cumin Can be used ground or as whole seeds. One of the principal ingredients of a curry, cumin is also incorporated into baked items as well as bean and rice dishes. Found in the spice section.

Daikon A Japanese radish with a white root like a large white carrot. Makes a great soup base. Found in the produce section.

Edamame Soybeans Buy frozen. They are a wonderful snack. Found at most grocery stores.

Fennel Whole plant available fresh, seeds available dried. A vegetable with a bulblike base. Sweet, fresh fennel has a licoricelike flavor. The seeds from wild fennel are flat and used as a spice. Found in the produce or spice section.

Flourless Whole-Grain Bread Organic whole or multigrain flourless bread made from freshly sprouted live grains. Found at health food stores.

Fusilli A corkscrew-shaped pasta. Found in the pasta section.

Gingerroot Has a peppery, pungent taste. Use it ground in breads or fresh in Asian or stir-fried dishes. Found in the spice or produce section.

Gomasio A Japanese condiment.

Italian Parsley This parsley has flat leaves and looks more like cilantro than the classic curly-leaf parsley. The taste is similar to but more pronounced than that of regular parsley. It is medium green with multipointed leaves about ¾ inch wide. A natural breath freshener. Often used to balance garlic in a dish. Found in the produce section.

Jalapeño   A hot chile pepper, green in color and used to spice foods up. Found in the produce section.

Lentils   There are more than fifty varieties. Found in the grain/rice section or Indian markets.

Marjoram   Sometimes called sweet marjoram. A mild Mediterranean herb similar to oregano. Found in the produce or spice section.

Mirin   An Asian cooking wine made from sweet brown rice. Found in the Asian condiments section of most grocery stores.

Miso   A fermented paste made from soybeans and used as soup base and seasoning, believed in Japan to be strengthening to the blood, stomach, and intestines. Light misos can be used in place of dairy. Pastes are not to be confused with powdered misos, which are inferior in taste and practically devoid of nutritional benefits. Given miso's saltiness, it replaces any salt in food. Provides essential amino acids, B vitamins, calcium, and iron. Found in the chilled health food section or at health food stores.

Mushrooms   *White/Button:* These are small mushrooms and the most common variety.
   Cremini: These resemble white/button mushrooms, but they are darker and larger.
   Shiitake: These are oddly shaped and chewy in texture.
   Portobello: These are large brown round mushrooms, usually 2 to 5 inches in diameter.
   All mushrooms can be found in the produce section.

Nayonaise   A mayonnaise substitute made from organic soybeans. Found at health food stores.

Nori   This is a dried seaweed, ebony colored, paper thin, and crisp. It is used in sushi and sometimes marketed as wild nori. Found in the Asian section of markets.

Parchment Paper A sturdy, heatproof, stick-resistant paper that can be used to wrap fish for oven baking *en papillote* ("in an envelope"). Found in the baking section of most supermarkets.

Plum Tomatoes These are also known as Roma tomatoes. Ideal for cooking. Found in the produce section.

Rice Dream A great milk substitute made from rice. Found in health food stores and some supermarkets (often it is shelved, not refrigerated).

Rice Syrup A mild, sweet syrup with a flavor resembling butterscotch. It is made from rice and barley. Found in the condiments section.

Serrano Chiles Chile peppers that are small and very hot. They are orange in color. Found in the produce section.

Sorghum Sometimes called sorghum molasses. A sweetener with a smoky taste and thick texture. Found in health food stores.

Soy Cheese A cheese substitute made from soybeans. Found in health food stores.

Soy Margarine Contains liquid soybean oil, soybeans, salt, vegetable lecithin, and water. A substitute for butter in baking. Contains no cholesterol and has a lower ratio of saturated fat. Use non-hydrogenated whenever possible. If using partially hydrogenated, use only occasionally. Found at health food stores and in some supermarkets in the dairy section.

Soy Sauce (Light or Low Sodium) A salty sauce made from soybeans. Found in the condiment section.

Sucanat An evaporated, granulated juice of the sugarcane plant. Found in health food stores.

Sushi-Grade Ahi Tuna The best grade ahi tuna, usually very red in color. Found in the fresh fish section.

Tahini   A smooth paste made from hulled sesame seeds. It is very high in protein. Found in the condiments section.

Tamari   A salty, sweet, slightly tart type of soy sauce. Found in the condiment section.

Tarragon   An herb best used fresh. The flavor, chemically identical to that of anise, is pretty well lost in drying. Too pungent to be cooked in soups, but great added to practically anything else (sauces, chicken, fish). Found in the produce or spice section.

Toasted Sesame Oil   A dark cooking oil made from toasted whole sesame seeds. Found in the Asian condiment section.

Van's Waffles   Waffles made with no chemicals and no dairy. Found in the frozen food section of health food stores.

Vegetable Concentrate or Paste   A condensed soup or sauce base made from vegetables. Found in the spice section or canned soup section.

Wasabi Powder   A Japanese horseradish. This is an extremely hot powder used to make wasabi paste. In the Asian section of markets.

Water Chestnuts   White crunchy Chinese bulbs with a sweet and juicy flavor. Boil, roast, or use to make flour. These can be found in the Asian or canned food sections.

White Northern Beans   Found in the grain or canned food section.

Whole Wheat Flour   Made from whole wheat grain. Found in the baking aisle of health food stores and most large supermarkets.

Yellow Wax Beans   These are similar to green beans in shape and texture, but yellowish in color. They are sometimes called "wax beans." Found in the produce or canned section.

additional recipe categories

Cooking with Kids
Waffles, Pancakes, and Crepes (page 107)
Blueberry Breakfast Frappe (page 103)
Healthy Trail Mix (page 145)
TV Tray-l Mix (page 144)
EZ Sloppy Joes (page 226)
Boca Tacos (see Tofu Tacos, page 228)
Comfort Pasta (page 233)
Checca Pasta (page 258)

Cooking for One
Jessica's Breakfast Smoothies (page 102)
Tuna and White Bean Salad (page 186)
Grilled Snapper (page 197)
Honey Teriyaki Cod (page 198)
Sesame-Crusted Salmon (page 191)

Goody Two-Shoes
Chilled Tofu with Scallion-Citrus Marinade (page 128)
Savory Squash Soup (page 160)
Homemade Vegetable Stock (page 150)
Lusty Lentil Soup (page 161)

Chicago Diner's Miso Soup (page 159)
Cream of Broccoli Soup (page 155)
JAC's Carrot Soup (page 148)
Country Vegetable Soup (page 151)
Honey Teriyaki Cod (page 198)

I Can't Believe It's Not Dairy

Stuffed Zucchini (page 124)
Smoked Salmon Spread (page 143)
Fondue 2000 (page 133)
Cream of Watercress Soup (page 153)
Coconut Sorbet (page 300)
Our Favorite Chocolate Chip Cookies (page 304)
Killer Brownies (page 308)
Chocolate Mousse (page 309)
Tofu Cheesecake (page 316)

I Know I Shouldn't, but . . .

Blueberry Crunch Muffins (page 109)
Fettuccine with White Clam Sauce (page 217)
Caviar Pasta (page 267)
Truffled Mashed Potatoes (page 280)

Impress Your Guests

Wild Mushroom Bruschetta (page 116)
Olive's Tuna Tartare (page 120)
Stuffed Grape Leaves with Lemon Sauce (page 130)
Border Grill's Ceviche de Veracruz (page 121)
Tricolored Vegetable Pâté (page 134)
Smoked Salmon Spread (page 143)
Shrimp and Black Bean Lettuce Wrap (page 123)
Fondue 2000 (page 133)
Cream of Watercress Soup (page 153)
Rob's Ribollita (page 168)
Cioppino (page 170)
Smoked Salmon Salad with Cucumber and Pine Nuts (page 187)

Seared Tuna and Caramel Soy (page 190)
Olive's Grilled Marinated Tuna (page 193)
Bow-Tie Pasta with Salmon and White Beans (page 216)
Whole Roasted Fish with Fennel (page 196)
Baked Golden Trout (page 195)
Baked Salmon with Sun-Dried Tomato Crust (page 199)
Coconut Shrimp with Curried Hummus on Wonton Squares (page 126)
Oven-Roasted Asparagus with Hazelnut Vinaigrette (page 270)
Tofu Cheesecake (page 316)

Leftover Potential
Joe's Black Bean Spread (page 140)
Tricolored Vegetable Pâté (page 134)
Tuscan White Bean Dip (page 142)
Summer Wrap (page 122)
Upside-Down Garlic Chicken (page 220)
Linguine with Red Clam Sauce (page 218)
EZ Sloppy Joes (page 226)
Rich Man's Stew (page 242)

Mass Appeal
Classic Bruschetta (page 117)
Smooth and Chunky Salsa (page 137)
Guacamole (page 138)
Upside-Down Garlic Chicken (page 220)
Tarragon Chicken (page 222)
Porcini Risotto (page 252)
Rich Man's Stew (page 242)
Our Favorite Chocolate Chip Cookies (page 304)
Chocolate Mousse (page 309)

Old Favorites
Waffles, Pancakes, and Crepes (page 107)
Cornmeal Flapjacks (page 105)
Sweet Potato Hash Browns (page 106)

Zucchini Bread (page 114)
Banana Bread (page 113)
TV Tray-1 Mix (page 144)
Stuffed Mushrooms (page 118)
Joe's Black Bean Spread (page 140)
Smooth and Chunky Salsa (page 137)
Guacamole (page 138)
Joanna's Gazpacho (page 158)
Linguine with Red Clam Sauce (page 218)
MaryAnn's Meat Loaf (page 239)
Super Bowl Chili (page 238)
Manicotti (page 235)

One-Dish Wonders
Soy Cheese and Mushroom Frittata (page 108)
Swiss Chard and Country Bean Soup (page 164)
Cioppino (page 170)
Rob's Ribollita (page 168)
Linguine with Red Clam Sauce (page 218)
Shepherd's Pie (page 236)
Castilian Rice (page 243)

Prep Now, Eat Later
Border Grill's Ceviche de Veracruz (page 121)
Joe's Black Bean Spread (page 140)
Stuffed Mushrooms (page 118)
Summer Wrap (page 122)

Quick and Easy
Jessica's Breakfast Smoothie (page 102)
Blueberry Breakfast Frappe (page 103)
Tuscan White Bean Dip (page 142)
Grilled Snapper (page 197)
Honey Teriyaki Cod (page 198)
Sesame-Crusted Salmon (page 191)

Mussels Sautéed with Tomato (page 206)
EZ Sloppy Joes (page 226)
Boca Tacos (see page 228)

Restaurant Madness
Polenta French Toast (page 112)
Olive's Tuna Tartare (page 120)
Border Grill's Ceviche de Veracruz (page 121)
Olive's Grilled Marinated Tuna (page 193)
Coconut Shrimp with Curried Hummus on Wonton Squares (page 126)
Grilled Portobello Mushroom with Sautéed Oyster Mushrooms (page 136)
Baked Salmon with Tomatoes, Olives, and Capers (page 200)
Steamed California Mussels (page 207)
Poached Salmon with Sherry-Shallot Mayonnaise and Black Beans (page 212)

Spread It Around
Guacamole (page 138)
Spicy Guacamole (page 139)
Joe's Black Bean Spread (page 140)
Tuscan White Bean Dip (page 142)
Smoked Salmon Spread (page 143)

Worth the Effort
Maple Danish (page 110)
Stuffed Grape Leaves with Lemon Sauce (page 130)
Tricolored Vegetable Pâté (page 134)
Wild Rice and Soy Chicken Salad (page 188)
Chicken with Tarragon (page 222)
Fettuccine with White Clam Sauce (page 217)
Coconut Shrimp with Curried Hummus on Wonton Squares (page 126)

Tasters' Top 10s

MaryAnn's
Asparagus Shiitake Mushroom Risotto (page 250)
Must-Have Macaroons (page 307)

Bow-Tie Pasta with Smoked Salmon and White Beans (page 216)
MaryAnn's Meat Loaf (page 239)
Tuna and White Bean Salad (page 186)
Olive's Tuna Tartare (page 120)
Creamy Daikon Soup (page 156)
Wild Mushroom Polenta (page 246)
Swiss Chard and Country Bean Soup (page 164)
Caviar Pasta (page 267)

Lorin's
Seared Tuna and Caramel Soy (page 190)
Olive's Tuna Tartare (page 120)
White Bean Pasta (page 263)
Porcini Risotto (page 252)
Our Favorite Chocolate Chip Cookies (page 304)
EZ Sloppy Joes (page 226)
Maria's Porcini Pasta with Pine Nuts (page 261)
Rich Man's Stew (page 242)
Fondue 2000 (page 133)
MaryAnn's Meat Loaf (page 239)

Lizzy's
Linguine with Red Clam Sauce (page 218)
Caviar Pasta (page 267)
Rich Man's Stew (page 242)
Whole Roasted Fish with Fennel (page 196), using striped bass
Creamy Daikon Soup (page 156)
Cilantro Corn Chowder (page 152)
Olive's Tuna Tartare (page 120)
Spicy Cold Soba Noodles (page 257)
Farfalle Funghi (page 260)
Porcini Risotto (page 252)

Bryony's
Salad Greens with Fresh Cucumber Dressing (page 178)
Thai Coleslaw (page 277)

Hunter's Tofu (page 232)
Our Favorite Chocolate Chip Cookies (page 304)
Upside-Down Garlic Chicken (page 220)
Guacamole (page 138)
Smooth and Chunky Salsa (page 137)
Must-Have Macaroons (page 307)
Shrimp and Black Bean Lettuce Wrap (page 123)
Stuffed Mushrooms (page 118)

Inara's
Guacamole (page 138)
Smooth and Chunky Salsa (page 137)
Shrimp and Black Bean Lettuce Wrap (page 123)
JAC's Carrot Soup (page 148)
Linguine with Red Clam Sauce (page 218)
Bow-Tie Pasta with Salmon and White Beans (page 216)
MaryAnn's Meat Loaf (page 239)
Brussels Sprouts with Vinegar-Glazed Onions (page 275)
Orange Cake with Carob Glaze (page 312)
Mexican-Style Rice Pudding (page 301)

index

Books by Marilu Henner: sources for the photographs

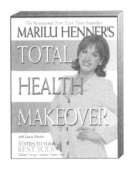

MARILU HENNER'S TOTAL HEALTH MAKEOVER

ISBN 0-06-098878-9 (paperback); ISBN 0-06-109828-0 (mass market); ISBN 0-694-51927-8 (audio)

With irrepressible enthusiasm and humor, Marilu presents practical advice on diet myths, toxic foods, mood swings, food combining, and her unique, flexible, down to earth 10-step life plan. With *Marilu Henner's Total Health Makeover* you can free yourself from diets and disease-causing toxins, boost your energy, lower and maintain your weight, and change your outlook in as little as three weeks.

THE 30 DAY TOTAL HEALTH MAKEOVER

Everything You Need to Do to Change Your Body, Your Health, and Your Life in 30 Amazing Days

ISBN 0-06-103133-X (paperback)

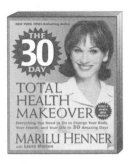

This inspirational how-to guide for total health living and your B.E.S.T. body in just 30 days includes day-to-day goals; strategies for success; recipes for breakfast, lunch, and dinner; shopping lists; exercise ideas; and what to feed the kids.

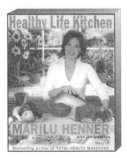

HEALTHY LIFE KITCHEN

ISBN 0-06-098857-6 (paperback)

Marilu Henner provides a delicious collection of healthy recipes that will help readers change their bodies and their lives forever. Created by Marilu and her favorite chefs from restaurants all over the world, these delectable breakfasts, lunches, dinners, desserts, and snacks will raise healthy cuisine to a new level of taste and ease. There is even a "healthy junk food" section for converting naughty treats into nutritious recipes.

I REFUSE TO RAISE A BRAT

ISBN 0-06-098730-8 (paperback); ISBN 0-694-52129-9 (audio)

Supermom Marilu Henner and renowned psychoanalyst Dr. Ruth Sharon provide simple and straightforward advice on how to raise secure, happy, and self-reliant children. *I Refuse to Raise a Brat* teaches readers how to distinguish between overgratification and love, break the pattern of overindulgence, and offer children the balance of frustration and gratification they need.

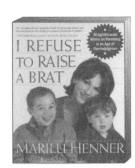

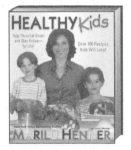

HEALTHY KIDS

ISBN 0-06-621112-3 (hardcover)

Marilu Henner believes that healthy food equals healthy children. In *Healthy Kids*, Marilu shows how the choice of diet for your child will influence his long-term health prospects more than any other action you may take as a parent. This essential guide shows parents that food provides the building blocks for a strong and healthy body, and giving your child the energy needed to learn, play, and grow.

Available wherever books are sold, or call 1-800-331-3761 to order.